I0846330

Balance Exercises for Seniors

Carson Robertson DC
Nina Russin

Alpha Dog Marketing LLC
4955 S Alma School Rd#10
Chandler, AZ 85248
robertsonfamilychiro.com

Base-Level Standing Exercises to Develop Proprioception

Nobody likes working on exercises they are not very good at. We all want to work on things that we enjoy and feel that we do a great job with. Many of the exercises and stability work are difficult and challenge your system. *It challenges all of the things you are not very good at, for a very good reason.* You have balance issues because the system is compromised.

Over time you will notice improvement in your ability to perform these exercises. You will be able to do them longer and with better control. Eventually you will fatigue, but it will take longer to hit your failure point. **That is an improvement.**

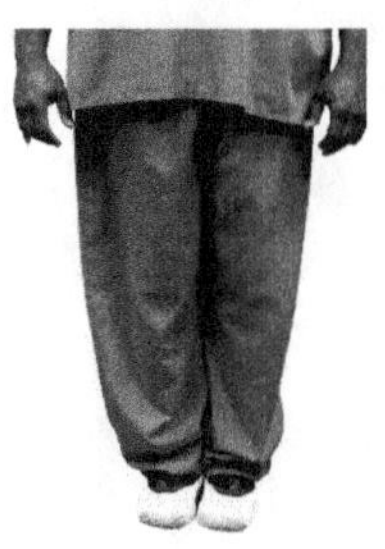 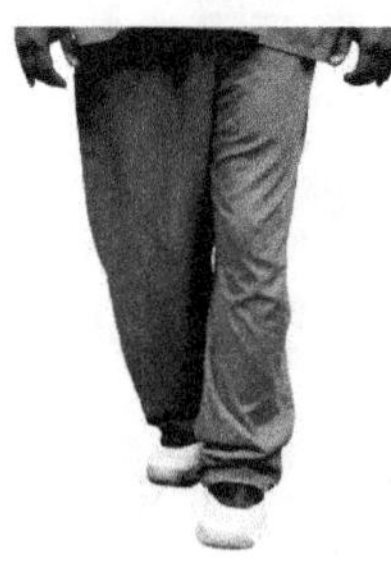 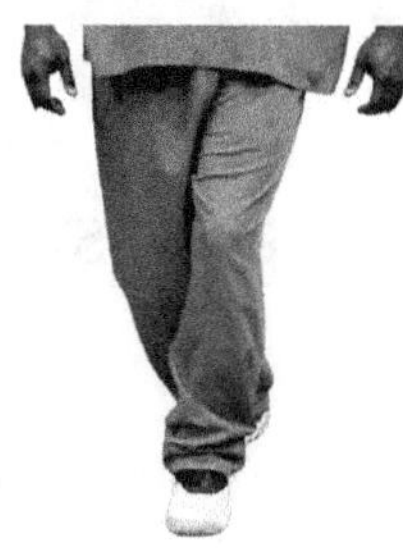 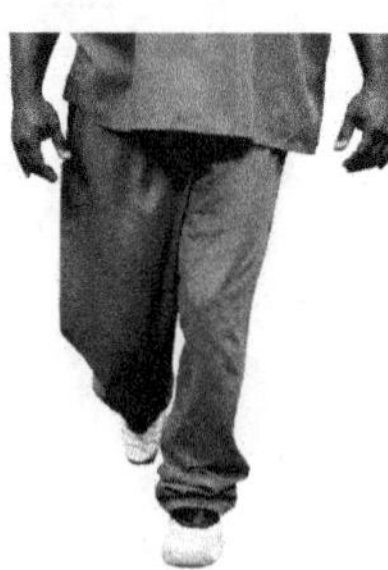 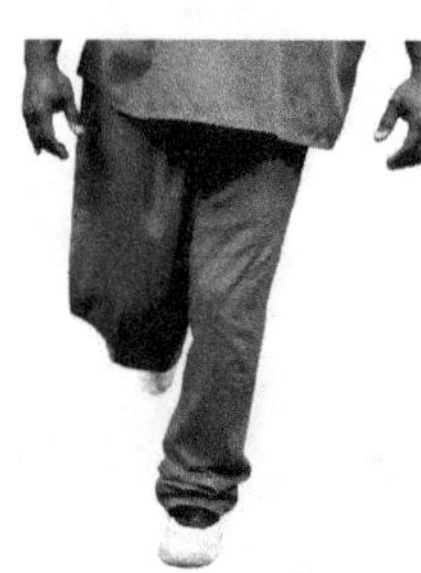

| **Together** | **Modified Tandem** | **Tandem** | **Single leg toe down** | **Single leg** |

The simplest of standing exercises is tandem stance, where you have one foot in front of the other like you're walking on a tightrope. For many people this is the initial exercise that they can properly perform. If you're having weakness and feel like you can't stay balanced in this position, then that's a sign of significant proprioceptive loss.

To make this exercise a step harder, close one eye. At this point we're losing input from our eyes, which helps with our stability. By losing a little bit of depth perception, it requires your body to listen to the ankle, knee, and hip joint receptors to keep stable.

Many people become very eye dominant for their proprioception. They stopped listening to their foot, ankle, knee, and hip joint receptors. For long term improvement, you need to reactivate the joint proprioceptors. Closing both eyes makes the exercise much harder and is one of the fastest ways to engage this system and enhance your recovery (be safe when and where you close your eyes - no falling).

From the tandem stance we can progress to a single leg stance with the knee slightly bent. We want to maintain proper posture in the back and hips, which then require the lower leg, upper leg, hip, and back muscles to work together. Single leg stance is making several muscular and nervous systems work together. This may sound simple, but I think you should try it before reading the next paragraph.

Rule of Thumb:

You should be able to hold your single leg stance position for over a minute with your eyes closed.

Try standing on one foot and squatting. If you can't stand on one foot try it with two feet shoulder width apart.   As you lower yourself, you'll notice that at some point you will want to hinge forward. <u>The point of the hinge is a sign of your strength levels.</u>

You were probably only able to squat another six to eight inches before hinging forward. <u>This is your breaking point</u>. Past this point you are unable to stabilize the knee, pelvis, or back because of muscle weakness. Your body went to its usual compensation method of hinging forward: lowering your shoulders towards the ground without moving your hips anymore. And yes, you should be able to squat lower on one leg then you just did for this test.

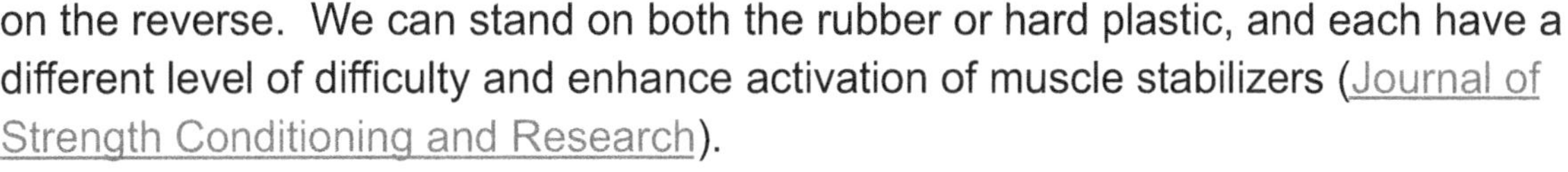

Further enhancement of the proprioceptive system involves unstable surfaces. There are a variety of unstable services that can be utilized. Anything soft and squishy, such as foam or rubber discs, works well. From here we can progress to more unstable services such as a wooden wobble or rocker board. Many people are familiar with BOSU balls, which have a rubber dome on one side and a flat, hard plastic side on the reverse. We can stand on both the rubber or hard plastic, and each have a different level of difficulty and enhance activation of muscle stabilizers (Journal of Strength Conditioning and Research).

Each of these exercises can be enhanced by closing one or both eyes. The more you require the body and brain to listen to the joint sensors in the ankle, knee, and foot, the faster you will improve.

All of these neuromuscular pattern exercises can be enhanced with a vibration unit. Vibration units continually knock you off balance, which requires the system to pull you back to neutral and stabilize. In the meantime you have been shifting to the opposite direction again and your body has to respond. The speed, amplitude, and frequency of vibration can be adjusted and each has a therapeutic advantage.

Rule of Thumb:

<u>Stimulus and Response.</u> The body responds to changing stimuli. If you want a reaction or different outcome, you need to challenge the body. The more stimulus we challenge you with, the faster you will respond. This is why level one exercises are great at the beginning but you need to progress past these to more challenging exercises.

Exercise balls can be utilized in many of the following exercises. Balance is more than just your feet and ankles. The pelvis, core, and back play an integral role in maintaining balance as you stand and walk.

Sitting on a ball makes the pelvis and core work together to keep steady. Adding arm movements or weights challenges the system even more. The exercises are always made easier with a wide base, two feet apart. Moving the feet closer together changes your stability and makes the body work harder. Eventually you can perform the same exercise with two feet tandem or on a single leg..

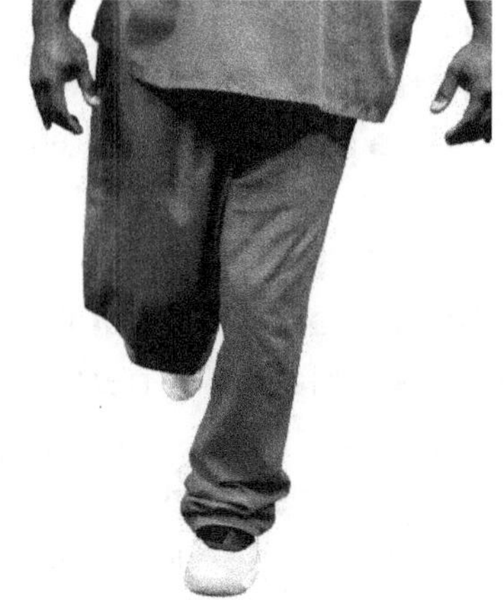

Most people are amazed at how difficult it is to maintain balance on a vibration plate. Every exercise is significantly harder and more challenging, which speeds your overall neuromuscular control and recovery.

Training on a vibration therapy machine is an excellent way to increase proprioception, blood flow, muscle strength, endurance, and stimulate muscle growth. The increased level of difficulty and entire body muscle contraction increases the effort and calories burned per hour, which can result in increased weight loss compared to performing the same exercises on the ground.

Our office utilizes vibration machines to quickly and efficiently develop neuromuscular patterns, strength, and endurance in injured areas.

Vibration, Unstable Surfaces, and Proprioception

Vibration plates have been around for many years and are used by all advanced or high-tech rehabilitation or sports training facilities. Athletes can utilize vibration therapy to further develop their proprioceptive sensors, enhancing their stability and neuromuscular control. Even a person who is in great shape can find vibration therapy difficult.

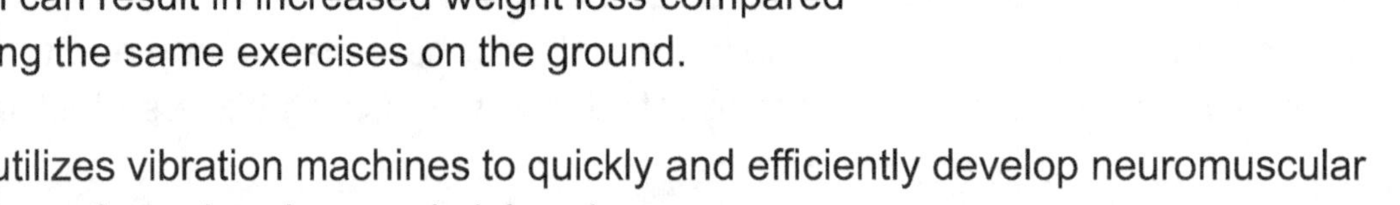

It's all about challenging the system and getting the body to respond. Every individual has his breaking point, and as a provider it is my job to identify your weakness and move you past it. We have had exceptional athletes get even better while challenging their one leg squat with their eyes closed. Of course they usually squat much lower and require more repetitions to reach their weakness. But the theory and process are the same.

The Exercise Progression
We always want to master the simpler exercise before progressing to harder exercises. Challenging the body's proprioception (balance) system increases your neurologic learning and accelerates your recovery.

The exercises always start with your eyes open. When you feel fairly steady, close one eye. This causes a loss of depth perception. Closing both eyes is significantly harder. Always perform eyes closed exercises in a safe environment when you can grab onto something for support, such as a wall or cane.

Challenge but don't overwhelm

This is a simple rule for balance exercises. Challenge the system but don't overwhelm. If your activity is overwhelming the body then it is not learning or adapting. The greatest improvement always comes with challenging your abilities with slightly harder exercises to make the system learn. The body does not learn when it is overwhelmed.

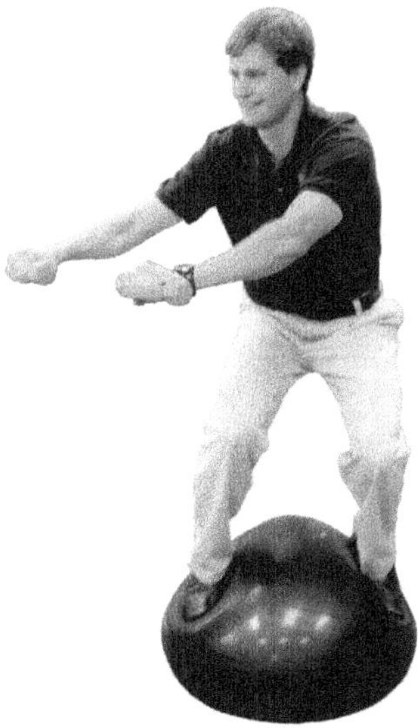

A long time ago I could stand on an exercise ball.

Balance & Stability Exercises

Sometimes you have to start in the basement and that is ok. It is not where you start, it is where you end. Please use the url links from the exercise title or QR code to see videos on YouTube.

<u>Door Frame Series</u>

The Door Frame series works to improve balance, along with how well the lower extremity works with the pelvis and core. In a door frame, start with two feet together. Keep your hands near the door frame to touch for support. Close one eye and try to keep steady, open the eye as needed or touch the door frame. With improvement close both eyes and maintain balance.

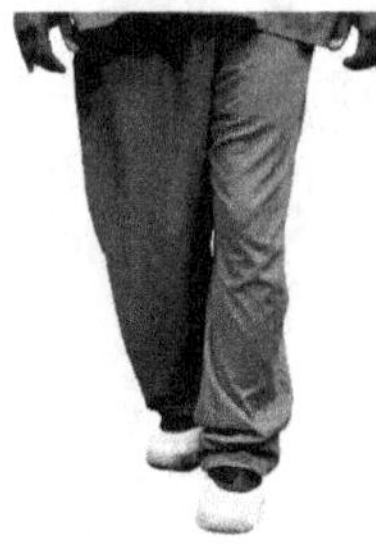

With improvement you can make the exercise more challenging by moving one foot backwards to a modified tandem position. The next hardest position is having the feet right behind each other, as if you were walking a tightrope. In each of these positions practice having both eyes open, one eye closed, and both eyes closed. No falling!

<u>**Single leg stance**</u>

Stand on one foot and stay steady. Your eyes and head should be facing forward with the shoulders and waist aligned. The knee should be pointing straight forward and not rocking inward. Your body weight should be distributed across the middle of your standing foot, while the foot arch is maintained and not flattening inward.

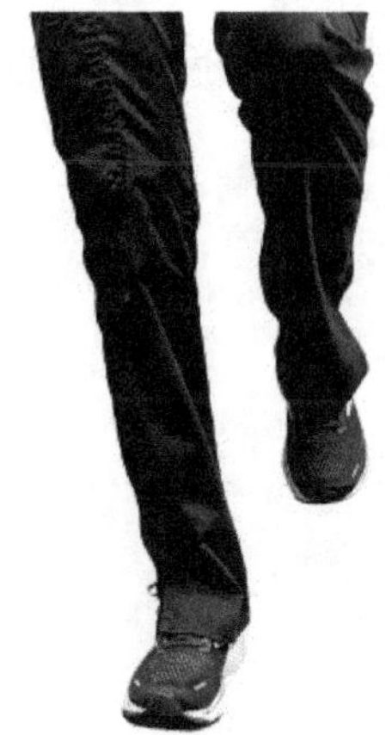

To make the exercises even harder, you can add slow squats or weights to the exercises. The exercises can also be performed on increasing unstable surfaces, such as a folded up towel, foam, BOSU ball, rocker board, wobble board, or vibration plate.

All of the exercises start on the ground and then progress to a more unstable surface.

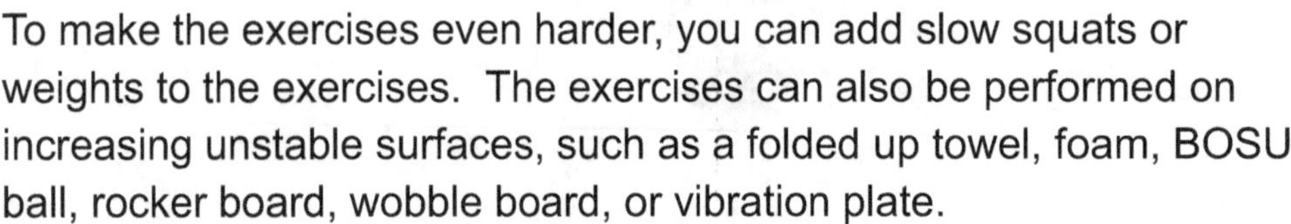

With the same foot positions as the door frame series this exercise will add rotation. Take the right hand and reach toward the left door frame. Try to hold the hand just above the frame without touching. Then slowly reach with the left hand toward the right door frame, focusing on slow rotation of the torso while maintaining balance. As in the door frame exercise, start with two feet together and then progress to tandem or single leg position. It is easier with both eyes open and then make the exercise harder by closing one eye. With improvement try closing both eyes and slowly rotating to the door frames.

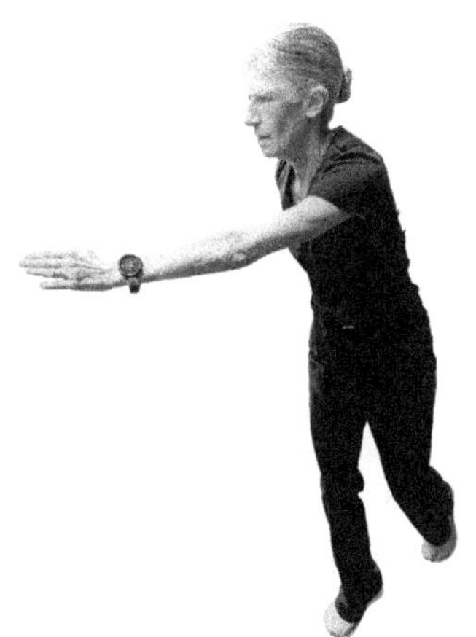
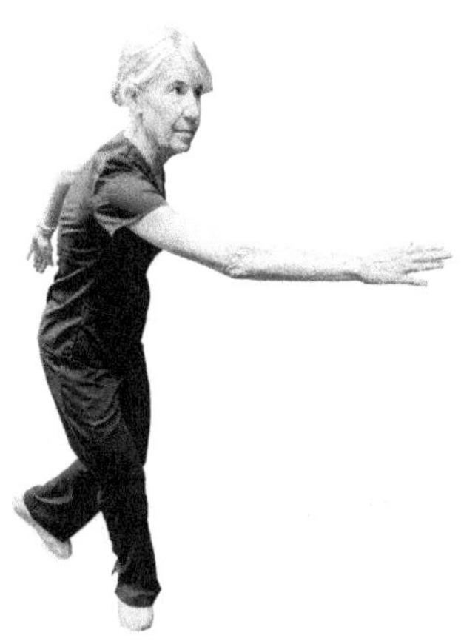

45, 90, 180 Laying on Bench

Laying flat on your stomach, raise your leg while keeping the knee straight. The movement should come from extending your hip and not rolling your pelvis. Perform 10 repetitions with the right leg before 10 repetitions with the left. Next, keeping the knee straight and toes pointed toward the floor, move the foot to the side abducting the hip. You will feel more muscle activation on the side of your glutes. Once again, perform all 10 repetitions before switching legs.

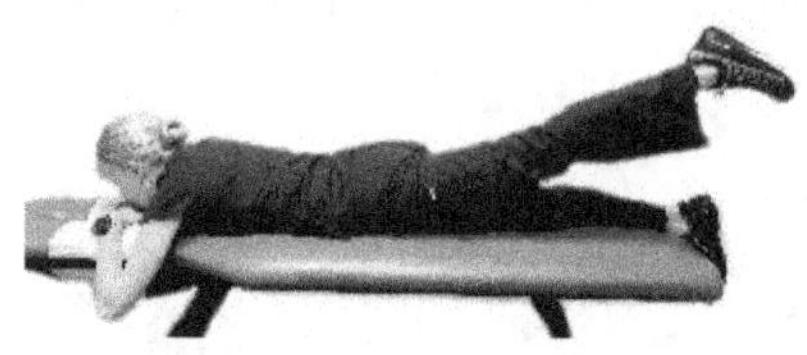

The last part of this exercise is to lift your foot at a 45 degree angle in a linear line. This is the hardest of the three for most people. Only go as far as you can without straining or rotating your femur. Build up to 3 sets of 10 on each leg. To make the exercise harder, go through the movements with a resistance rubber band.

Standing Hip Exercises: Door Frame (45° / 90°/ 180°)

Standing hip exercises challenge the hip stabilizer while incorporating balance activities. We begin the exercise inside a door frame for stability by keeping our hands on the frame, and with improvement taking the hands off. The exercises incorporate three planes of movement. The exercise takes the leg to the side, backwards, and at a 45 degree angle.

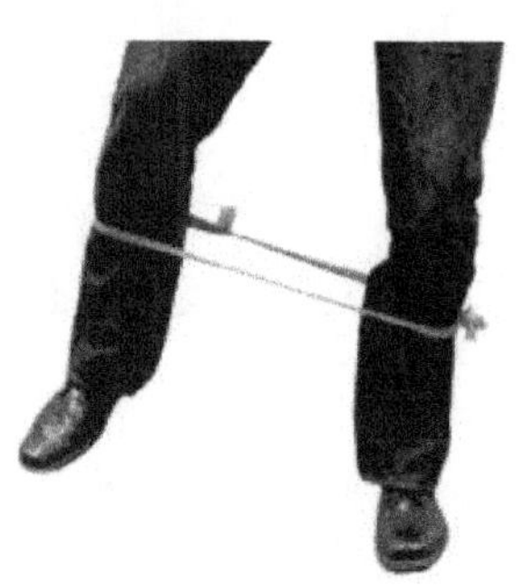

The three positions work all of the glute muscles; max, medius, and minimus muscles while incorporating balance and pelvic stability. With improvement an exercise band can be added to make the exercise more difficult.

Single Leg Hip Abduction - Toe in / Out/ Straight

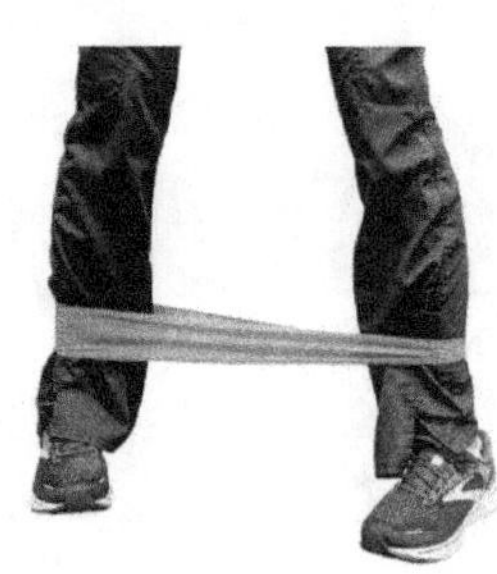

Standing on one foot, abduct the raised leg to the side. Concentrate on slow and steady leg movements while maintaining balance. A rubber band can be added around the legs to make it more difficult.

Calf Raises

Standing with two feet shoulder width apart, slowly raise your heels off the ground as you keep your balance. Then slowly lower your heels back to the ground. Initially start with two feet, then progress to single leg when your strength improves.

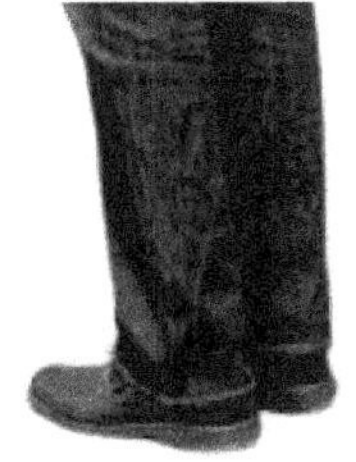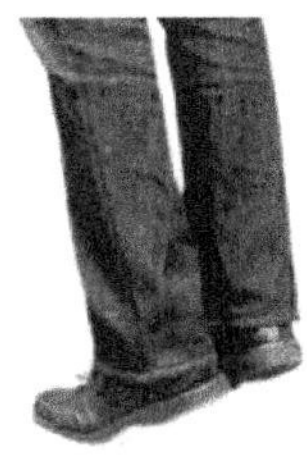

Step Ups

Start with a three-inch aerobics step or balance foam. Stand behind the step and practice stepping forward and up the step while keeping your knee pointing forward. Try not to shift your body weight to the side, compensating for hip and knee weakness. Over time and improvement, increase the height of the step. Increase stride length to add difficulty.

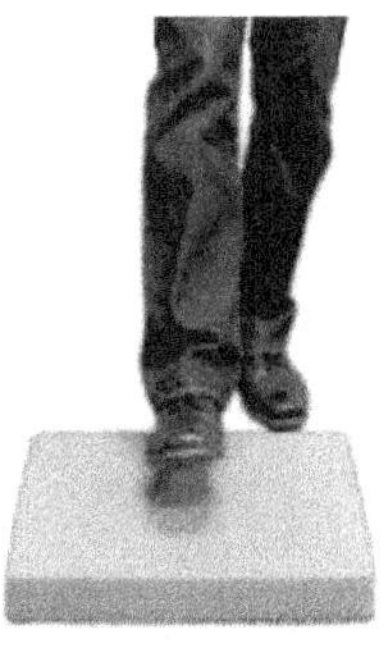

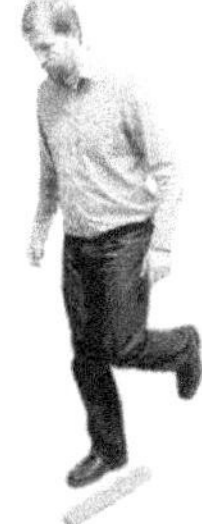

Side Steps Across Foam

Start by standing on your right leg with the left held slightly above the ground. Step to the left and shift weight to the left leg. Then lean back to the right and raise your left foot off the ground. Once you are steady on your right leg, repeat the exercise 10 times per side.

Side Step Ups

Just like it sounds. Step onto the step sideways. Focus on keeping your waist as level as possible and controlling your torso rock. Step both up and down the steps each direction.

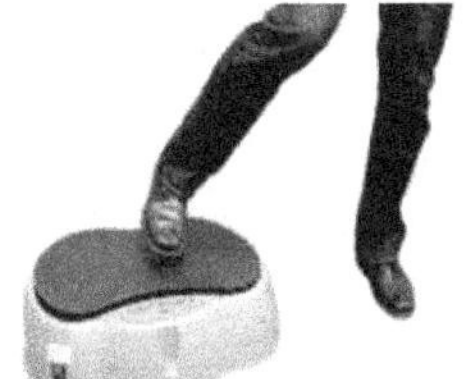

Square Dance

Stand on your right leg with the left held slightly in the air. Keeping all your weight on the right foot, reach the left behind you and tap the ground without supporting any body weight. Then reach the leg forward and tap a point in front of your right leg.   Next reach back and to the left, tapping the ground, then reach forward and to the left. Think of tapping the corners of a square. Repeat 10 times on each leg.

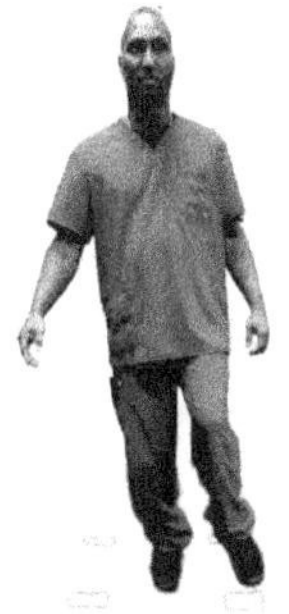

Once you have become comfortable with the square dance exercise, begin crossing behind and in front of your body. When standing on your right leg, your left foot will tap a point behind and to the right of your body. Likewise, when standing on your left leg, tap a point in front and to the left of your body.

These exercises are challenging your knee and hip balance while increasing stabilization strength and endurance.

Clock Exercise

Think of the face of a watch, not a digital clock. Standing on one foot with the raised foot held behind you, rotate as far as you can counter clockwise. Keeping your hands at your chest and your back straight, squat down as far as you can, maintaining form and balance. Tap your toe onto the ground. Like the hands of a clock, you are probably at the 8 or 9 o'clock position.

Slowly rotate clockwise one position and squat again. Work through all the positions of a clock dial that you can, and then repeat going counter clockwise.

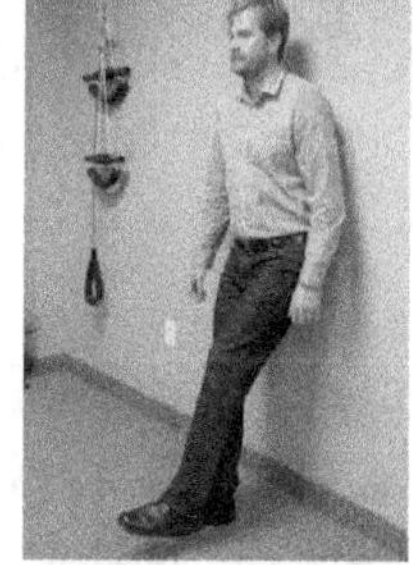

Single Leg Posterior Hip Bumps

Stand six inches from a wall on your right leg, with your left held in front. Slowly move backward until you fall into the wall, and then push yourself off the wall with your hips. Once you regain a steady balance on one foot, repeat the exercise. As you improve, move further from the wall.

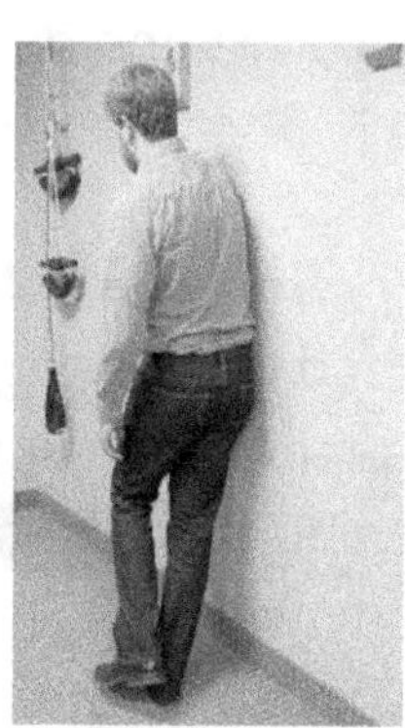

Side Hip Bumps

Similar to the posterior hip bumps. Standing with your hip facing the wall, fall to the side. Push off the wall with your hips and regain your balance. You will need to start closer to the wall compared to the posterior hip bump exercise. Hip bump exercises can be made more difficult by standing on an unstable surface or with your eyes closed.

Start by leaning with your back against the ball, and the ball positioned in the small of your back. Your legs should be straight and feet slightly forward, so that your knees don't move forward of your toes when you squat.

Start with squatting a few inches at a time. As you feel stronger and more comfortable work towards a half squat. If you feel comfortable, work towards a full squat. Slowly squat down until your knees form a ninety-degree angle, then return to a standing position. Start with one set of ten and work your way up to two-to-three sets.

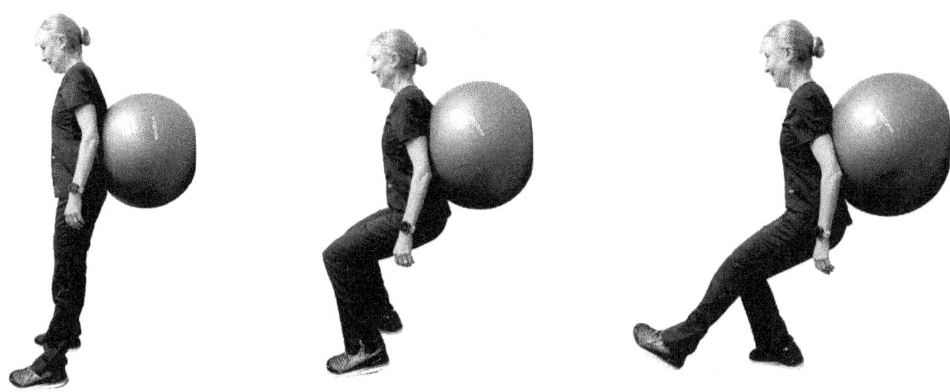

To make this exercise more challenging, place your two feet together and squat down. Eventually you can change your foot position to a tandem or single leg. Changing the feet position is similar to the door frame series in that it is a progression to one foot.

During a squat if the tibia (lower leg bone) is tipping backwards toward the wall it will place a greater emphasis on glute contraction. Likewise when the tibia is forward the quadriceps are more activated.

To focus on the glutes instead of the quads. Move your feet further away from the wall, which does feel awkward but you are leaning backwards into the wall. Start with squatting a few inches to engage the glutes and hip and slowly begin to squat lower and lower.

Sit to Stand

Getting out of a chair requires hip and leg strength. There are ways to increase hip and quadriceps strength by using the chair. We can keep our feet two feet apart and place our hands on our knees to help push and stabilize. A second step is to move the feet closer together. With improvement push off your leg with less force. The feet can also be staggered for the sit to stand.

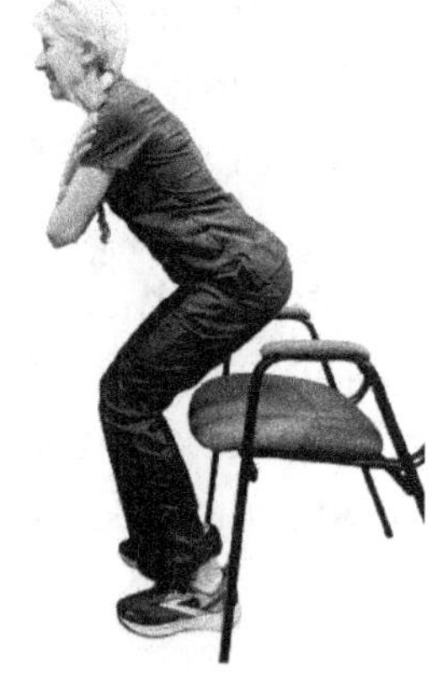

Another way to build strength is from a standing position, try and lower yourself to the chair without using your hands. You will feel yourself "plunk down" on the table. This is the point where the hip strength was unable to support the body.

Bird Dog / Quadruped

Start out in the quadruped position on the mat, with both hands and knees on the floor. Slowly extend the right arm straight forward and left leg straight back. Your arm, torso and leg

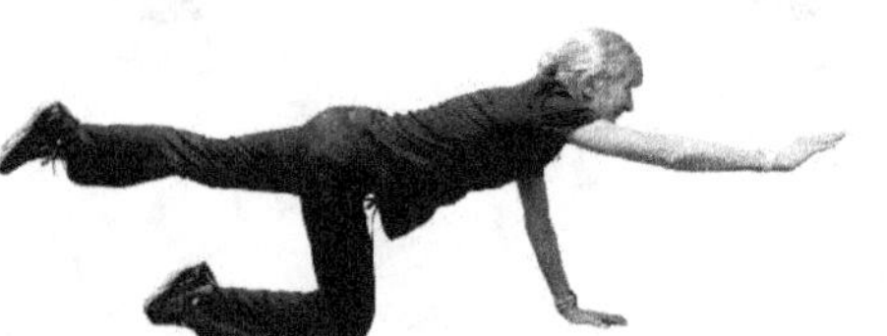

should form a straight line. Bring the arm and leg back down to the floor and reverse. Ten arm and leg lifts on each side constitute one set.

Thoracic Rotation Quadruped

An easy thoracic rotation exercise to add into the routine. This is a beginner exercise and a good stepping stone to harder thoracic rotation exercises. Like any of the quadruped exercises, narrowing the base stance will make it a little more difficult by challenging the stabilizers.

Start on your back with knees bent and feet shoulder width apart. Slowly raise your waist toward the ceiling, trying to pick your pelvis up toward the ceiling but not extending your back. The idea is to create a straight line from your shoulder through the waist and to the knees. Concentrate on slow and steady movements up and down, keeping the waist level at all times. Avoid swaying or tipping the pelvis during the movement.

Bridging exercises start with two feet apart and then move to two feet together. Then move to a position with one foot on top of the other and next, on one leg with the lifted knee bent. Finally, the lifted knee is kept straight. The progression is mastering 3 sets of 10 with two feet apart before moving on to two feet together. Then progress to one foot on top of the other for 3 sets of 10 before moving onto single-leg position.

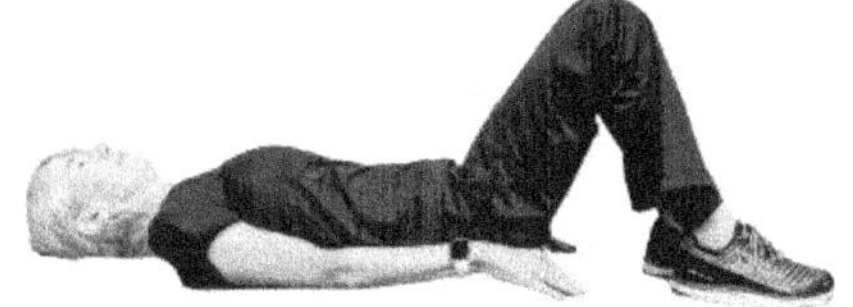
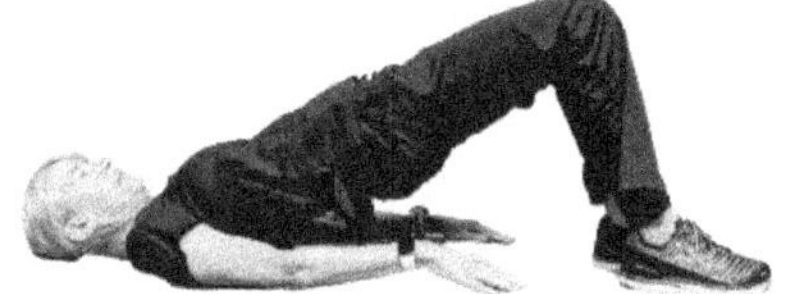
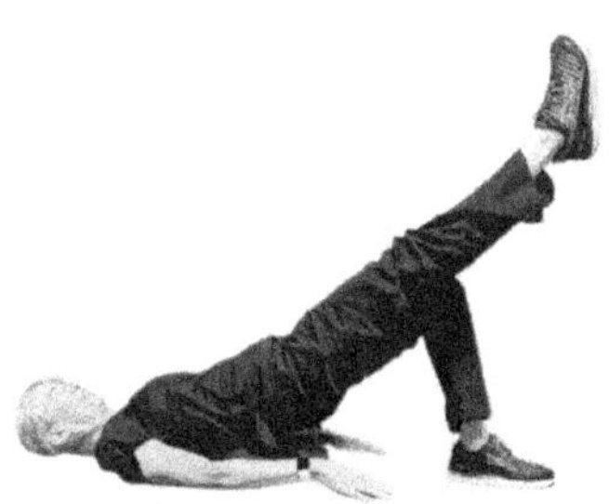

Glute Bridge on an Exercise Ball

If you have mastered the glute bridge on the floor, you can make the exercise more challenging by performing it on an exercise ball. We recommend having a spotter the first time you try this to make sure that the ball doesn't slip out from under you. If you don't know somebody who can help out, place the ball against a wall to make it more stable.

Start by rolling out on the ball so that the ball is supporting your head, neck, and upper back. Your feet and knees should be shoulder width apart. Cross your arms across your chest. Now lower your butt towards the floor and raise it back up to a table top position. Repeat 10 times for a set. To make this exercise more challenging, try it with your feet and knees together. Rest one foot on top of the other to make it more challenging still. For an advanced version, perform the bridging with one foot on the ground and the opposite leg straight out in front of you.

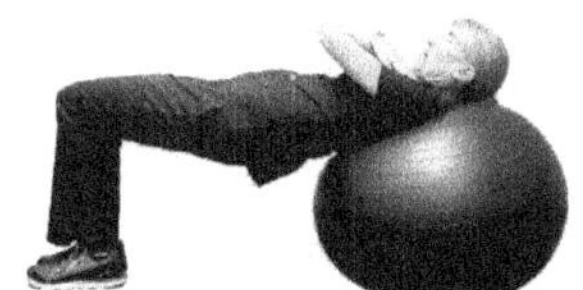
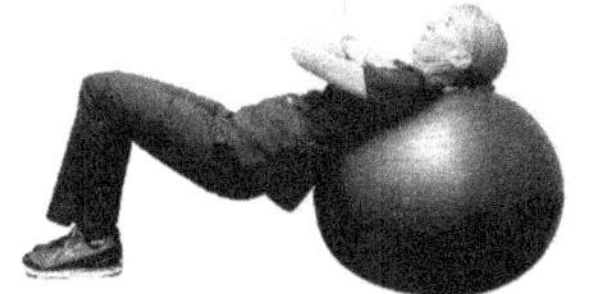

Slow Walk Resistance

With a mild resistance rubber band around your ankles, begin walking in a straight line. Do not move fast. Focus on slow, controlled movements and maintain resistance for most of the exercise. The walk can be exaggerated with a swinging leg to the side, or a monster-type walk.

Duck Walks

Side to side walks are used to increase lateral hip, knee and ankle strength. Place a resistance band around your ankles and keep tension on the band throughout the exercise. Initially, move slowly stepping with the lead leg to the side and even more slowly as you bring the trail leg back toward the middle. Don't lose tension on the band as the trail leg nears the lead leg. There are three positions for duck walk:

1. Toes pointing straight forward the entire time.
2. Toes pointing inward the entire time.
3. Toes point out the entire time.

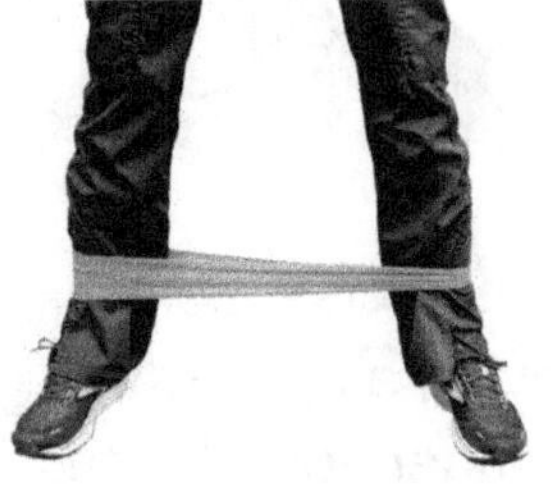 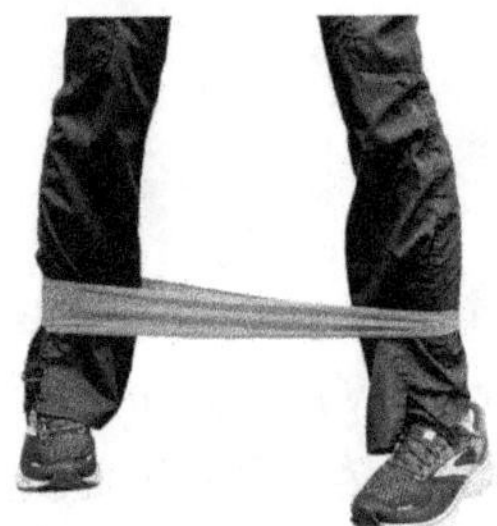 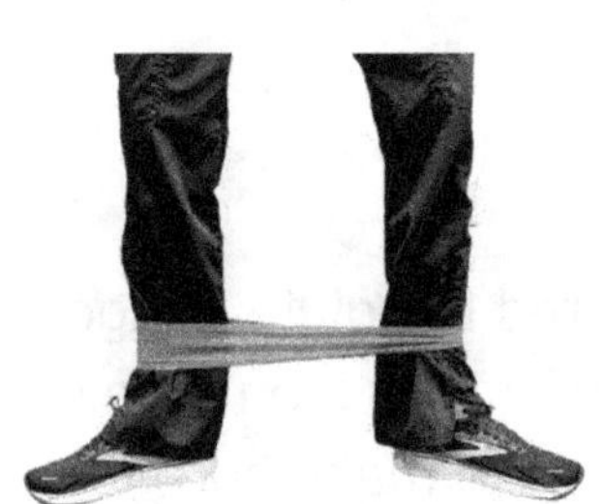

Lateral Hip Strength Exercises with Slider & Rubber Band

The slider helps to focus on slow and controlled movements and the rubber band adds resistance to build strength and endurance.

Move the foot as if reaching for the numbers on a clock and work all the way around. Turning the foot also subtly changes the exercises as you move through the progression. The exercise can be made more difficult by holding a weight, a stiffer rubber band, or using an elevated platform.

Lunge Step with Sliders

Step down and lunge exercises can progress to using a step and a slider. Start with small step and slider movements and progress to larger movements with improvement. Slide as if touching all the numbers on a clock to develop full hip and pelvic range of motion and strength.The slider helps to slow the movement and enhances the exercise into all directions of movement.

Start with slow and controlled movements and increase the stride with improvement.
The exercise can be made more difficult by using a taller step, adding a weight, or using a rubber band.

Medicine Ball Woodchopper

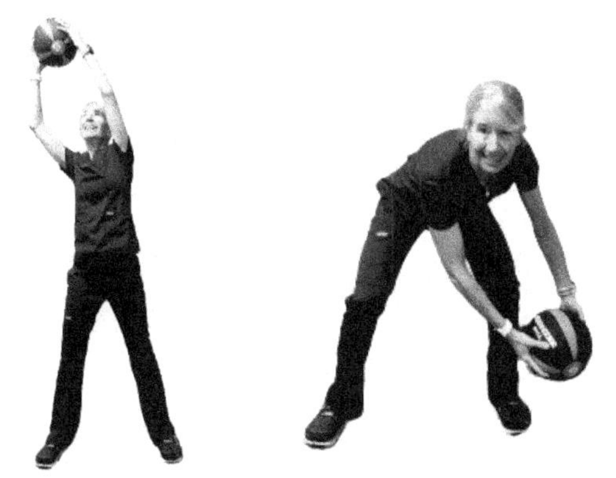

Begin standing with feet shoulder width apart, holding the medicine ball straight out in front of you. Reach up and to the right with your arms extended, then bring the ball down and to the left, bending

your knees for a full range-of-motion. Your back should remain straight and flexed slightly forward. Keeping the arms straight, bring the ball up on the left-hand side and fully extend your arms,   now swing it down and to the right, bending the knees as you go. Ten "chops" in each direction is one set.

Start with your arms at your sides. If you feel unsteady, do this exercise near a wall, table, or sturdy chair to hold onto. Lunge forward with one leg. Glide the waist forward and slightly lower until you feel a stretch. As with squats, it is not necessary to do a full, deep lunge to benefit from this exercise. Move the forward leg back to the starting position and lunge forward with the opposite leg. Start with one set of 10 and work your way up to two sets (image 1).

Initially, do not lower your waist all the way to the ground. Perform the exercise in a stable and controlled manner. With increased leg and hip strength, you will be able to go lower and perform more repetitions. A variation is to raise the opposite arm in the air and extend the torso backwards (image 2). Another option is to rotate the torso and arm (image 3). Do not force or strain with the torso or arm variations.

To make it easier, the lunge can be performed with a knee on the ground for stability. A pillow or towel can be placed under the knees for comfort (images 4, 5, and 6).

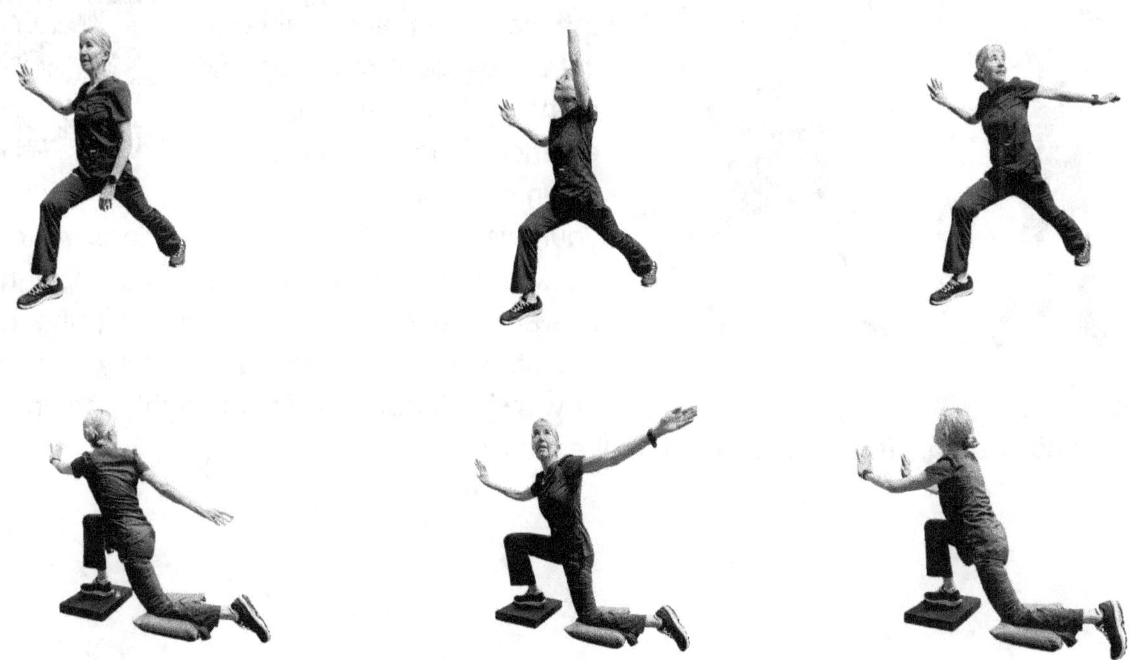

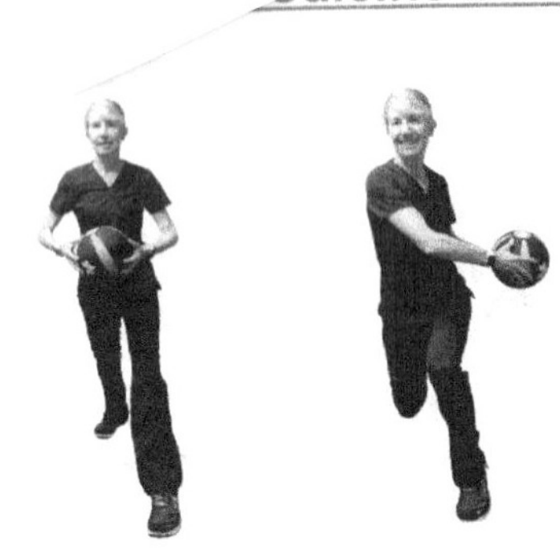

Medicine Ball Twist

Stand with your feet slightly apart, holding the medicine ball in front of you. Lunge forward with the left leg, while swinging the medicine ball to the right. Return to the standing position while moving the ball back to midline. Repeat for a total of ten lunges and twists on each side.

A reverse lunge is also a great exercise for hip and lower extremity strength. The exercise is performed with a step backwards and then squat. Lunges can focus on quadriceps or glute strength depending how they are performed.

Dot Drill

The dot drill actively moves in all directions. Placing five dots on the ground, similar to the patterns on dice, step from dot to dot. Step with one foot first and then bring the other foot the position, and then move to the next position.

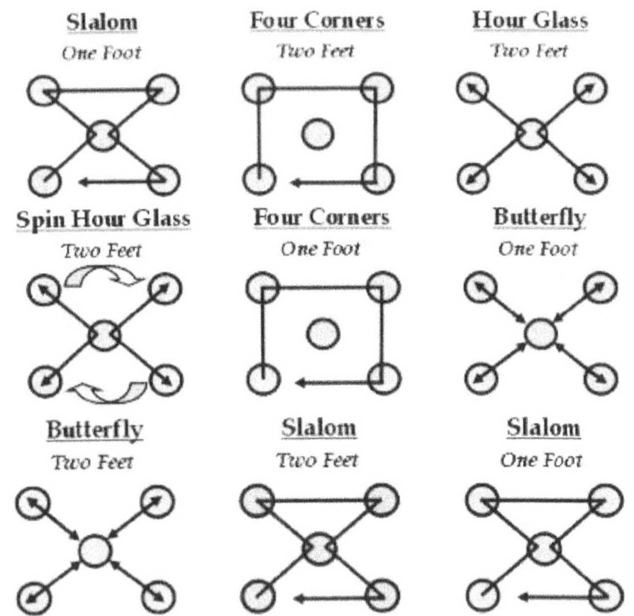

Ball Sitting Exercises

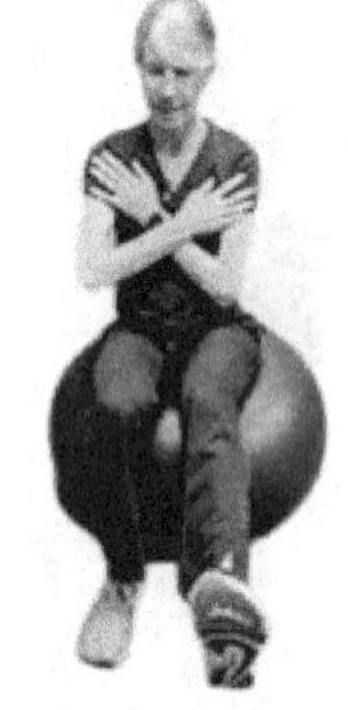

<u>Seated Leg Raise</u>

Sit on the ball with your arms crossed. Slowly raise the left leg, lower it and then raise the right leg. Repeat 10 times with each leg for a set. Eventually you can add a weight to hold in front of you or to the side for added difficulty.

<u>Seated Ball Rotational Twists</u>

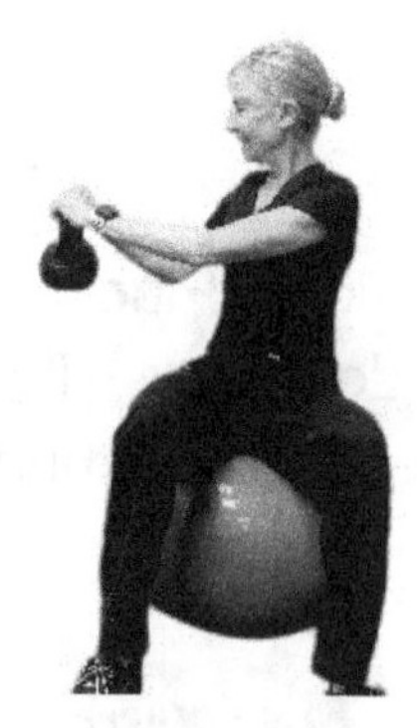
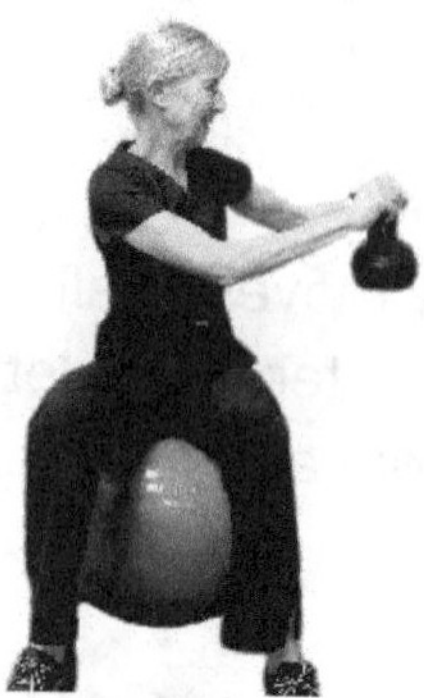

Sitting on the ball with feet shoulder width apart, slowly rotate the torso to the left. Pause for a few seconds and then rotate toward the right, pausing at the end range of motion. These exercises can be made more difficult by moving your feet closer together or holding a weight in your hands. Eventually the weight can be held in front of the torso during the movements.

Seated Ball Chop

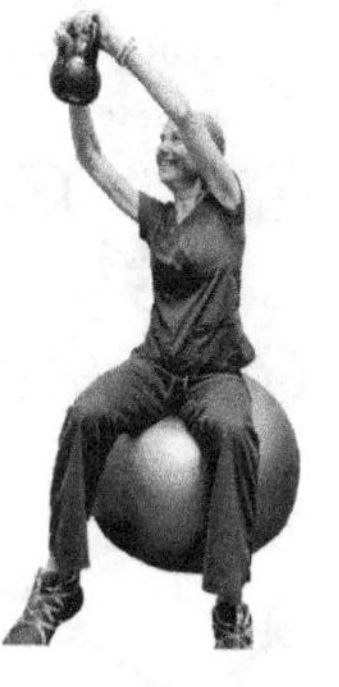
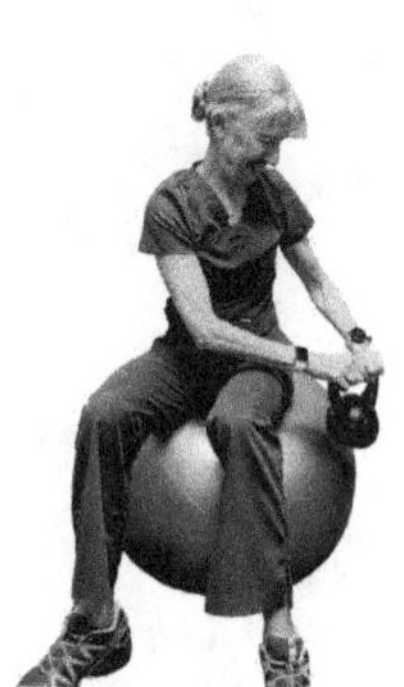

A variation of the medicine ball woodchopper exercise, sitting on the ball with hands in front. Reach up and to the right with arms extended, and then reach down to the left. A medicine ball or small weight can be used for added difficulty. Perform this exercises in both directions.

A 2004 study published in *Spine Journal* demonstrated that hip stabilization was also compromised in patients with chronic low back pain. In the study, "Hip Strategy for Balance Control in Quiet Standing is Reduced in People with Low Back Pain;" individuals with chronic low back pain were four times more likely to fail testing of postural stabilization and core stability.
https://www.ncbi.nlm.nih.gov/pubmed/15014284

Although core muscle weakness is one of the problems leading to low back pain, glute weakness also contributes. Overactive hamstrings and hip flexors attempt to stabilize the pelvis and lumbar spine. Exercises that activate, engage, and coordinate the glute muscles with the core are necessary for long term improvement.

Medicine Ball Pull-over
Roll the ball out so you are supine with the exercise ball supporting your upper back. Hold the medicine ball between your hands and extend your arms straight up so the ball is above your chest. Keeping the arms straight, extend the ball so it is slightly behind your head. Then move the ball back to the starting position keeping the arms straight. Repeat nine more times for a set.

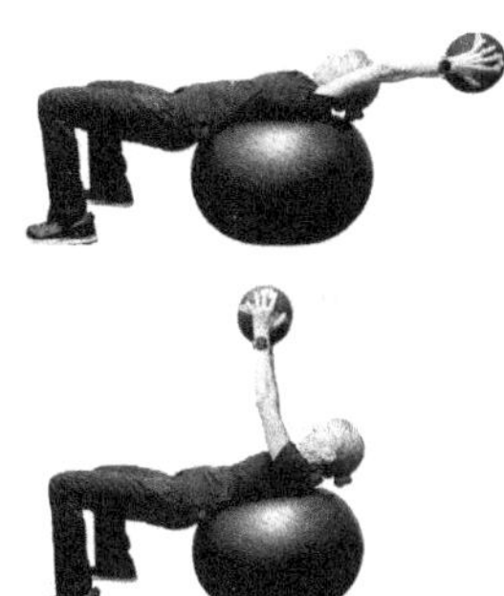

Bench Press on a Ball
Lie supine on the ball with the ball supporting your head, neck, and upper back. You may need to experiment a little bit to find the position most comfortable for you.

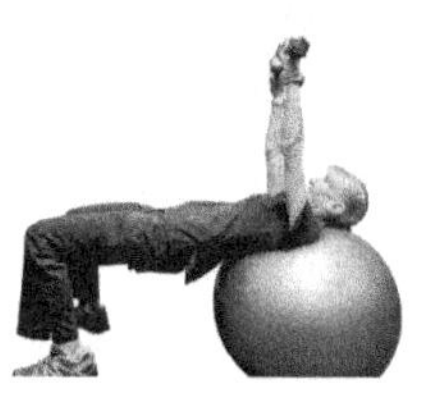

Use a set of dumbbells to do your bench press exercises on the ball. Because you are doing this on the ball, you should begin with lighter dumbbells than what you would normally use (remember, the ball makes this a lot more challenging).

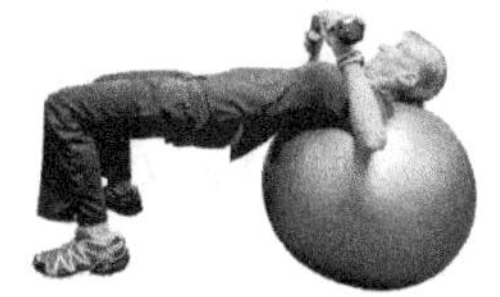

Lateral Raise on the Ball
You may have done similar exercises at the gym while standing or using a cable machine. In this version, you will start by sitting on the ball with a relatively light dumbbell in each hand. Your arms should be straight with the weights lowered as much as possible. Raise the weights up to shoulder height and lower them back down. Don't let the upper trap muscles take over; keep your shoulders relaxed.
A variation of this is a front lat raise, in which you
raise the dumbbells to shoulder height straight out in front of you.

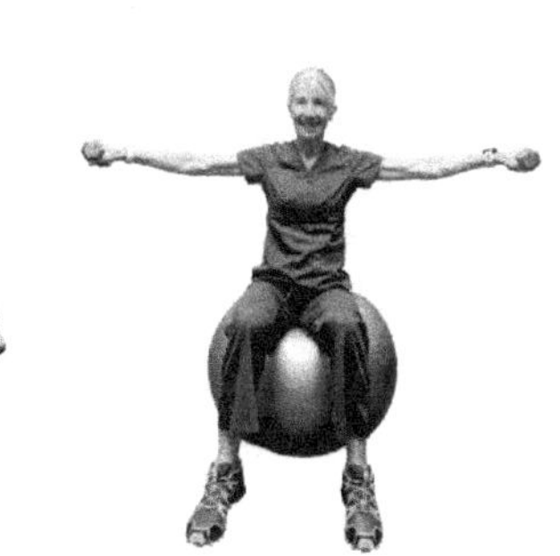

<u>FlexBar Shake</u>

Do this exercise while sitting on an exercise ball or standing. Hold one end of the FlexBar and extend your arm out to the side or out in front. Then shake the bar. This exercise will enhance your grip, upper arm, and shoulder strength. To make things more challenging, do woodchopper movements while shaking the Flexbar. Twisting at the waist to the right or left while shaking the FlexBar challenges the core.

A 2018 article published in the Journal of Physical Therapy Sciences, "Effects of Stabilization Exercise Using Flexi-bar on Functional Disability and Transverse Abdominis Thickness in Patients With Chronic Low Back Pain," evaluated the benefits of adding a Flexbar to core stabilization exercises. People performed 30 minutes of exercise three times per week for six weeks.
https://www.ncbi.nlm.nih.gov/pmc/articles/PMC5857446/

One group performed stability exercises by adding a Flexbar to further challenge proprioception and stabilization. While the control group performed the same exercises without the Flexbar. Adding the Flexbar increased stimulus to the deep spinal stabilizer muscles, producing greater improvement in functional stability and reduced pain levels.

Flexbar provides a similar stimulus to the upper extremity that standing on a vibration plate does for the lower extremity.

Many people think they need to lift heavy weights to exhaustion to gain strength and endurance, but that is not true. Functional workouts often provide greater benefit to people because they challenge the weakest muscle groups and neuromuscular control systems.

The TheraBand FlexBar is a great tool for developing arm strength and coordination. Rubber FlexBars come in different widths and stiffness, so you can use them to rehab an injury or to enhance your strength in a key area.

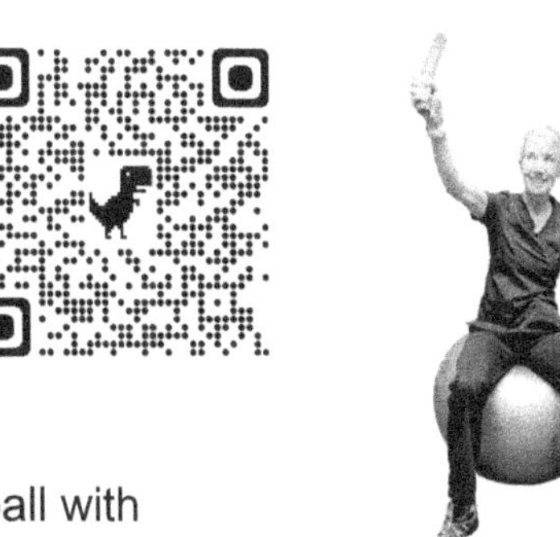

This exercise can be performed standing on the ground, foam, or unstable surface. Perform the exercises in tandem stance or single leg for added difficulty. Sitting on the ball with changing foot position also challenges the core and balance system.

Radial and Ulnar Deviation

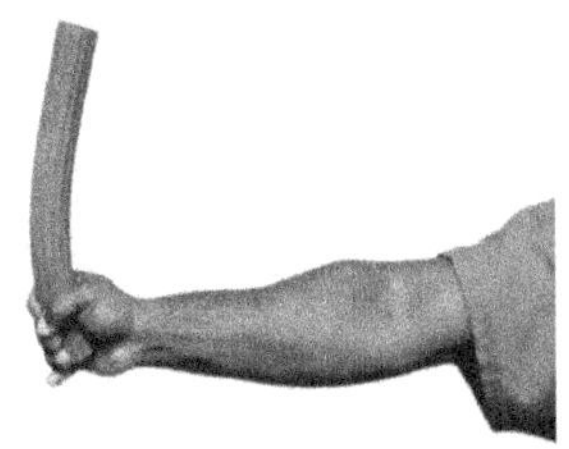
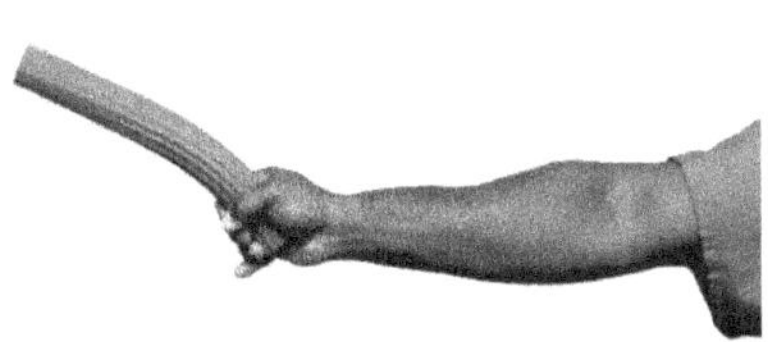
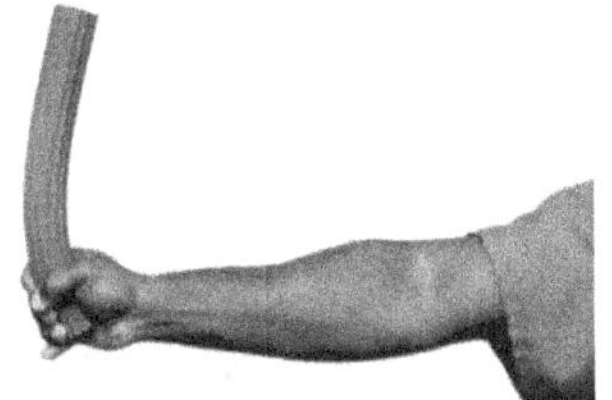

Pronation and Supination

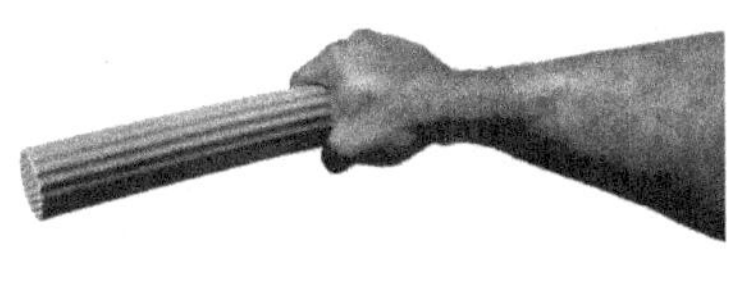
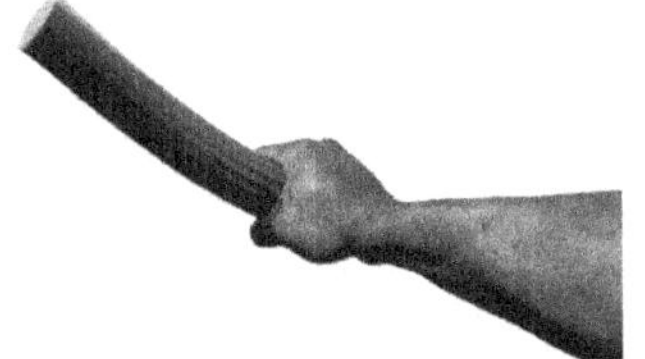
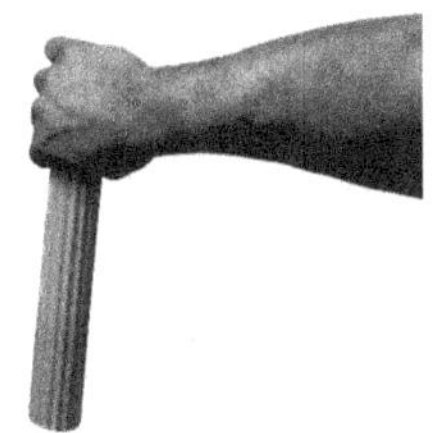

FlexBar Twist

Hold the end of the FlexBar in each hand, twist the bar in one direction and then back in the other direction.

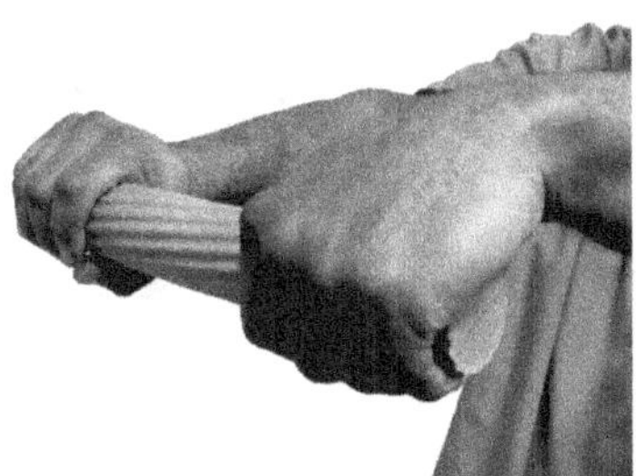
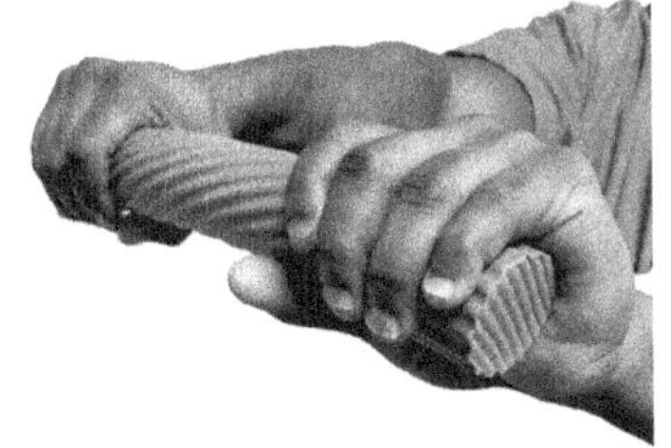

This video explains why we focus on the lower scapular stabilizers to improve the shoulder. Knowing the "why" helps patients focus on their form and continue doing the "boring exercises." I highly recommend you watch this video if you have shoulder pain.

External Rotation

Hold one end of the TheraBand in your hand. Your elbow should be bent, and your hand will be at your body's midsection. Keeping the elbow bent, rotate the band outward. Bring it back to the starting position and repeat 10 times for a set.

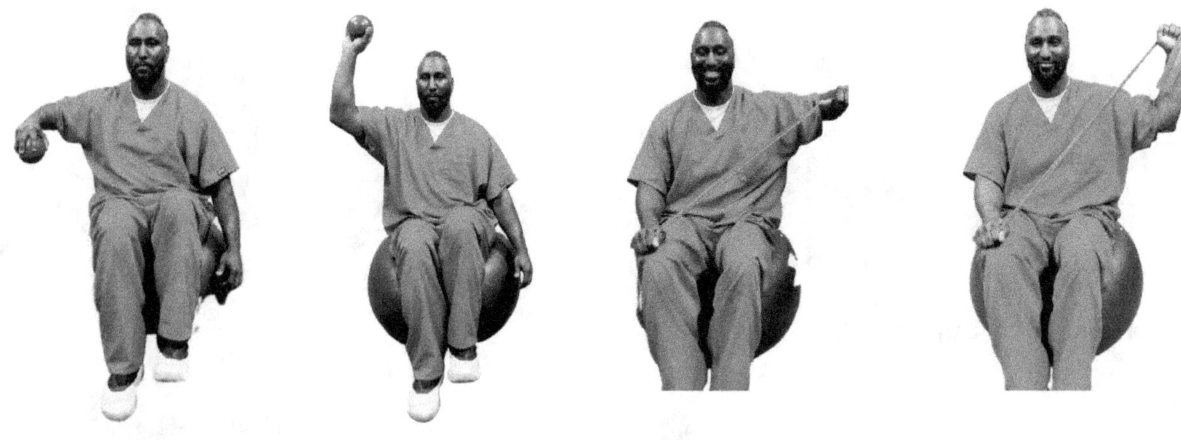

Internal Rotation

This is the opposite of the external rotation exercise. Start with the hand rotated away from the body and rotate it inward towards your midline.

Bilateral External Rotation

Hold one end of the TheraBand in each hand, keeping your elbows bent and upper arms next to your body. Your hands should be at your body's midline. Rotate each end of the band outward, then return to the starting position. Repeat 10 times for a set.

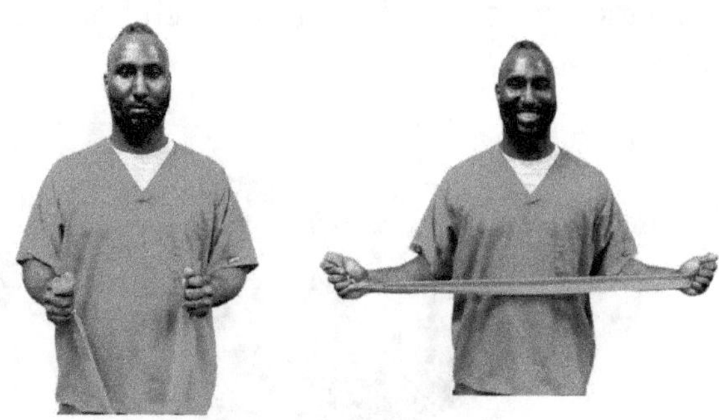

This exercise can be performed sitting on a ball or standing with two feet together or single leg. We use these exercises as a way to improve your balance while strengthening other parts of the body with a band or light weights.

Similar to performing the motions to the song YMCA, instead you will be performing YTWL. Repeat 3 times. The Y-T-W-L can be performed as a stretch. It can also incorporate bands and small weights as an exercise. It can be performed standing, sitting on a ball, or lying prone on a bench.

Y - Make a big Y with your arms with the elbows straight, and then pull the arms backwards until you feel a comfortable stretch. Hold for 10 seconds.

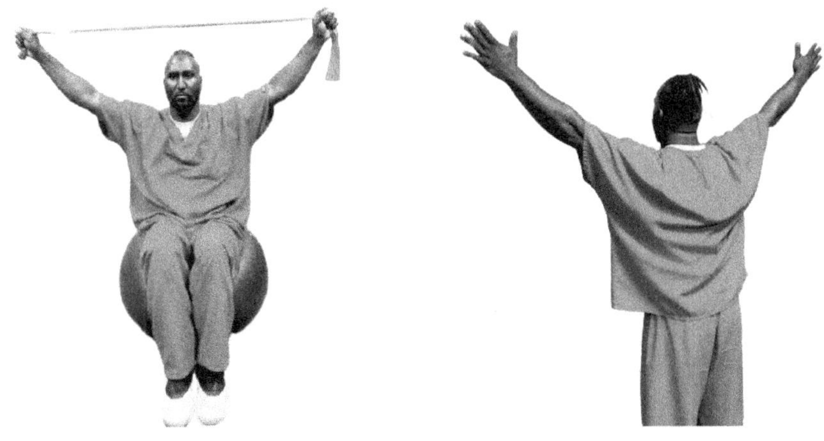

T - Lower your arms and form a T, once again pulling the arms backwards for a comfortable 10 second stretch.

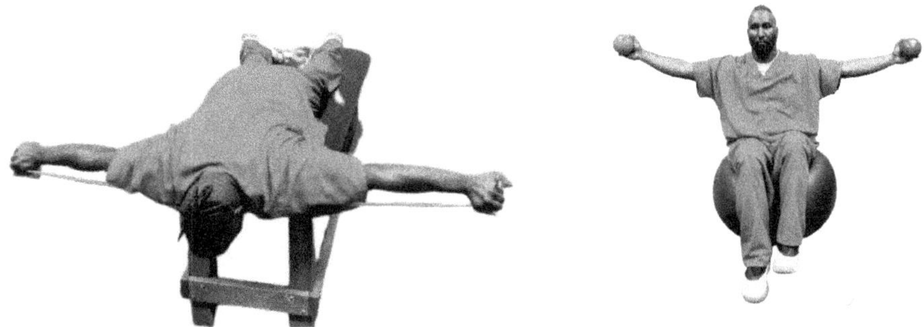

W - From the T position bend your elbows with them lowering toward the ground, form a W with your arms.

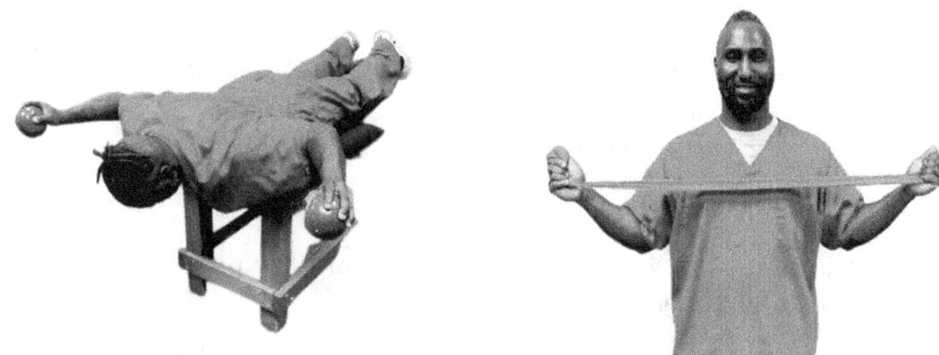

L - From the W position, lower your hands until a 90 degree bend occurs at the elbow. The elbow should be touching the torso. Stretch the hands backwards for 10 seconds.

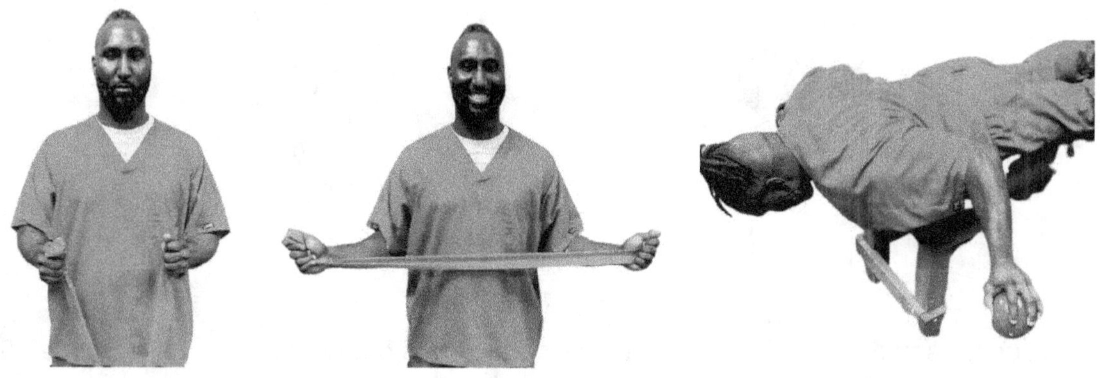

Y-T-W-L Band / Ball / Weight Exercise
Performing the **Y-T-W-L** with resistance exercise bands. Slow and smooth, concentration on keeping the scapula low. These are great exercises to focus on eccentric movements.

These are great exercises to slowly increase upper body strength, endurance, and joint stabilization in a pain-free zone. The ball is placed along the wall at various points. Pushing with a steady pressure produces an isometric force into the ball. With improvement, slow movements or rotations can be included. Think of Karate Kid with the wax on and wax off movements: slow and controlled.

Changing the hand position changes the muscle groups involved. Switch from having the palm of the hand on the ball to the back of the hand.

We can also improve balance with these exercises by shifting your feet from shoulder width apart to two feet together. Then try moving one foot backwards to a tandem position. It is quite a bit harder when trying to balance on one leg and perform the ball on the wall exercise. Try it.

Incorporating changing foot positions toward a single leg and performing ball on the wall exercises increases balance and coordination between the upper extremity, scapula, core, pelvis, and lower extremity.

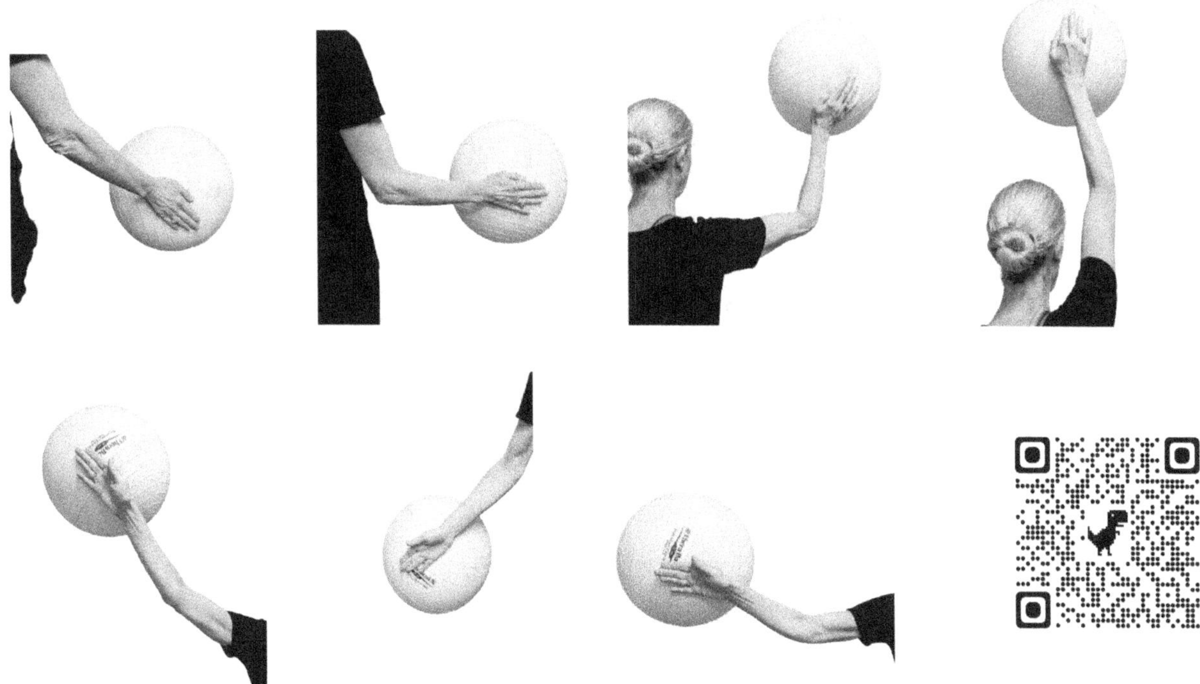

Place the ball on the back of your hand to strengthen the shoulder muscles in the back of your arm and scapula, click to watch instructions for the posterior shoulder muscles.

Balance and Chronic Back Pain

A person with chronic low back pain also loses balance and stability while standing and walking. For example, the ability to stabilize oneself when standing on one foot

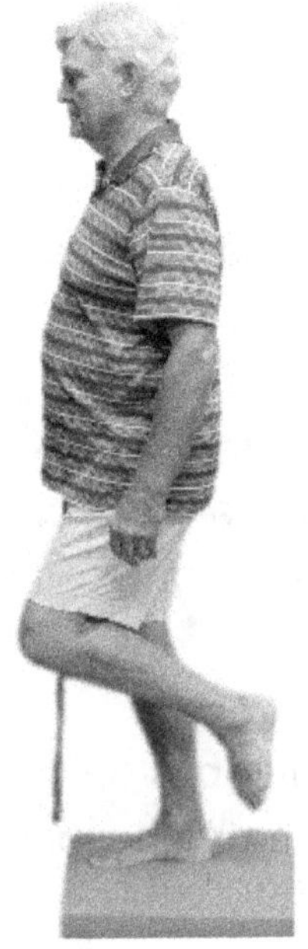

decreases with chronic low back pain. As a person's condition continues to deteriorate, the single leg stance stability worsens. The poor balance is a consequence of pain and poor proprioception from the low back facet joints, and weakness and loss of stability from the deep spinal stabilizer muscles.

This is not a new concept. A study published in 1998 in the journal *Spine* titled "One-Footed and Externally Disturbed Two-Footed Postural Control in Patients with Chronic Low Back Pain and Healthy Control Subjects: A Controlled Study with Follow Up" evaluated this principle.

The study concluded: "Postural stability is easily disturbed in case of impairment in strength, coordination, or effective coupling of muscles in the lumbar and pelvic area. Patients with chronic low back pain seem to experience impairment in these functions, which should be taken into consideration when back rehabilitation programs are planned." https://www.ncbi.nlm.nih.gov/pubmed/9794052

Building on the recommendations of the prior study, a 2018 study published in the *Journal of Exercise Rehabilitation*, "Comparison of the Effects of Stability Exercise and Balance Exercise on Muscle Activity in Female Patients with Chronic Low Back Pain," showed that back pain was reduced in both stability and balance exercise groups, through different mechanisms. https://www.ncbi.nlm.nih.gov/pmc/articles/PMC6323339/

A similar finding appeared in a 2018 study published in the *BMC Musculoskeletal Disorder Journal* titled "Postural Awareness and its Relationship to Pain: Validation of an Innovative Instrument Measuring Awareness of Body Posture in Patients with Chronic Pain." The study found that improving posture decreased spinal and shoulder pain. https://www.ncbi.nlm.nih.gov/pubmed/29625603

For this reason we combine traditional strengthening exercises with stability and balance exercises to reduce back pain and enhance spinal stability.

Abdominal Curl Up

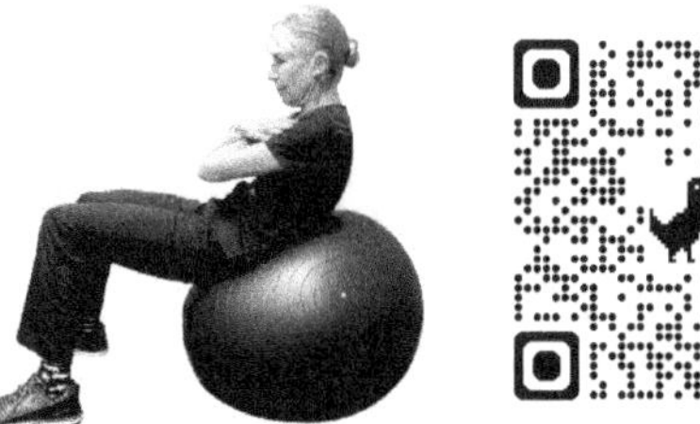

The ball should be positioned to support your lower and middle back. With your arms positioned so that your hands are supporting your head and neck, tighten abdominal muscles and curl up slowly. Return to the original (supine) position. To add challenge, twist while curling, first to the left and then to the right.

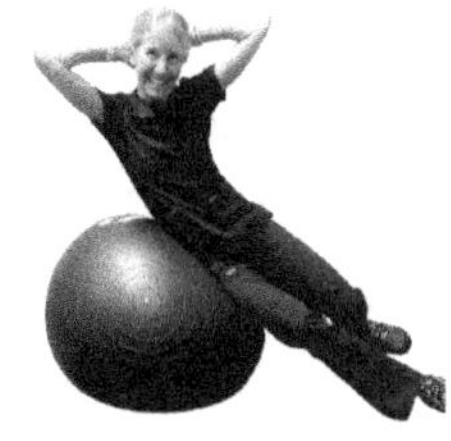

Lateral Curl Up

Start with your feet on the floor, lying on your side with the ball under your hips. You may want to prop one of your feet against a wall to anchor yourself. Curl up sideways, then lower back down to the starting position. Repeat for a total of ten lifts on each side.

Cross Crawl Ball

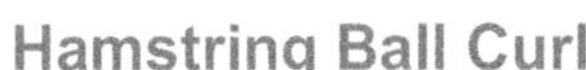

Start in a prone position with your hands and feet touching the floor and the ball under your trunk. Slowly lift the left arm and right leg off the floor and extend them so that they are aligned with the body (straight out to the front and back). Lower them back to the starting position and lift the opposite limbs. A set consists of 10 lifts on each side.

Hamstring Ball Curl

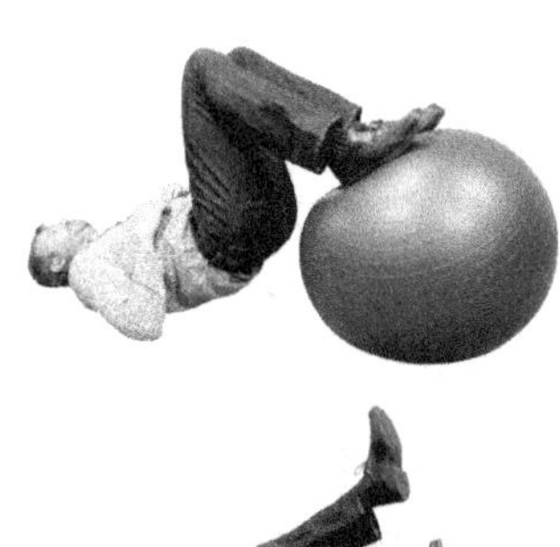
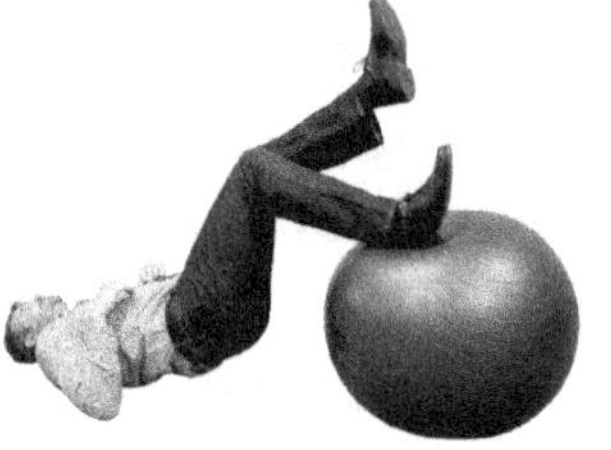

Laying on your back with two feet on an exercise ball, lift your waist into the air. Next, pull your feet into the ball and roll it toward your waist. The harder you pull into the ball, the more stress will be applied to the hamstring muscles. After you pull the ball as far as you can, extend your legs as you maintain pressure into the ball. The exercise can be performed with two feet or a single leg.

Foot & Ankle Exercises & Stretching

Ankle and foot motion
With your ankle start by pointing your toes up as far as you can and then pointing down. Then point the toe inward as far as you can and then outward.

Alphabet motion
Pretend your big toe is a pen and write the letters of the alphabet. You can write capital and lowercase letters. This is not the most exciting exercises in the world, to keep yourself entertained after a while try writing words or song lyrics.

Resisted ankle motion with bands
We use the rubber band to increase strength and endurance. Use the same motions of ankle and foot motion exercise, but with the added difficulty of the rubber band. Start with the foot in neutral and then move through the motions of flexion, extension, inversion, and eversion. Slowly move away from neutral, and then even slower move back to neutral.

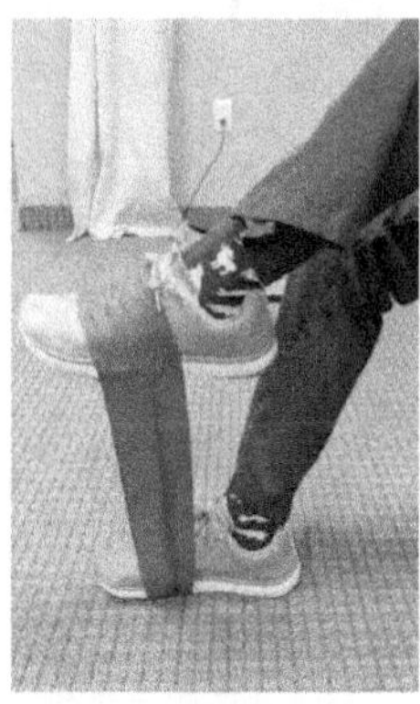 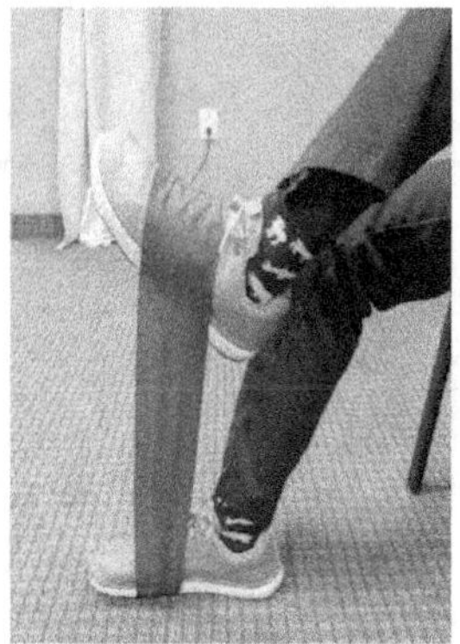 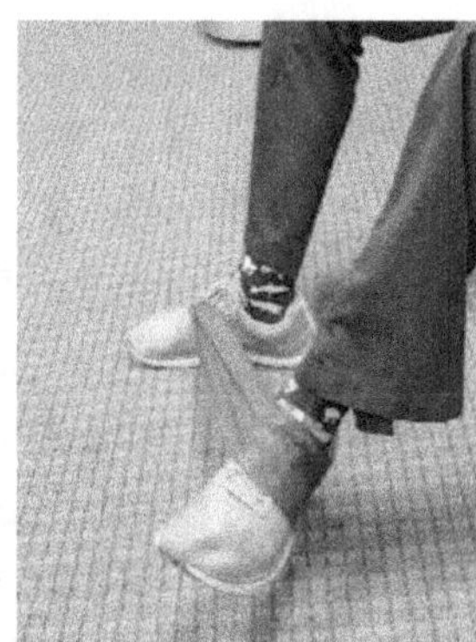 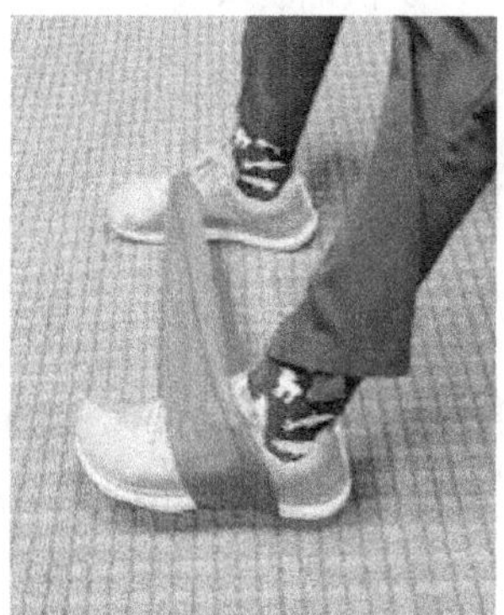

Towel grabs
With your toes on a towel flex and scrunch your toes, pulling the towel toward you. This can also be adapted to picking up golf balls, or anything that causes toe flexion.

Toe spreading
Toe spreading involves spreading your toes away from each other, which can be repeated to fatigue. It is not hard, it just takes practice for some. This strengthens the little muscles that control the toes and foot.

Foot Doming

While standing on one foot, lift your arch creating a dome. Hold this position for a few seconds and then relax. Gradually hold the position for longer periods of time.

Lower Leg

The calf stretch can be performed standing with the foot flat on the ground, on a step, or with a foot rocker (prostretch). Having the knee straight or bent will focus the stretch on the two different calf muscles: gastrocnemius and soleus.

Place the left foot behind you with the heel on the ground. Glide your waist and body weight forward until a stretch is felt in the calf (image 1). Hold onto a wall for extra support if needed. Performing the same stretch with a bent knee will focus more of the stretch onto the soleus muscle.

Using a prostretch or calf rocker is another variation. Place your right foot onto the rocker and push the heel toward the floor. Watch the Calf Stretch with Pro Stretch explanation.

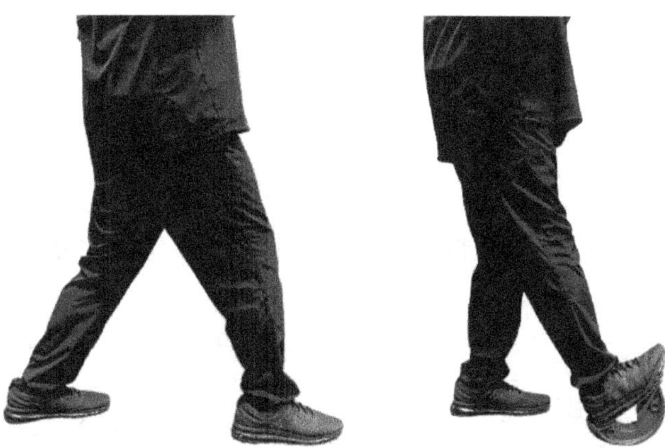

The front of the lower leg can be stretched by either pulling your ankle backwards or resting it on a bench with the toe pointed (image 1). Sitting on the heel will create a greater stretch (image 2).

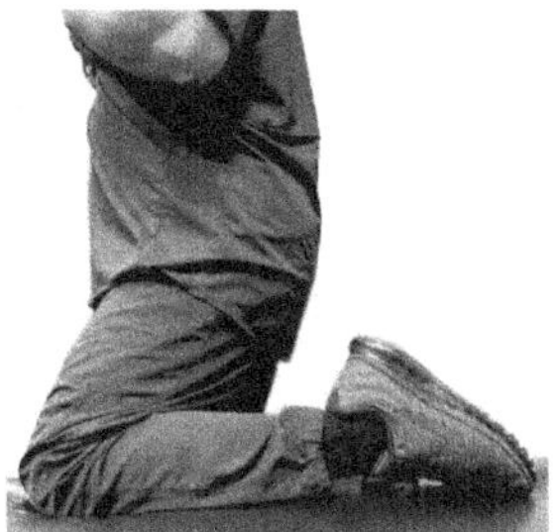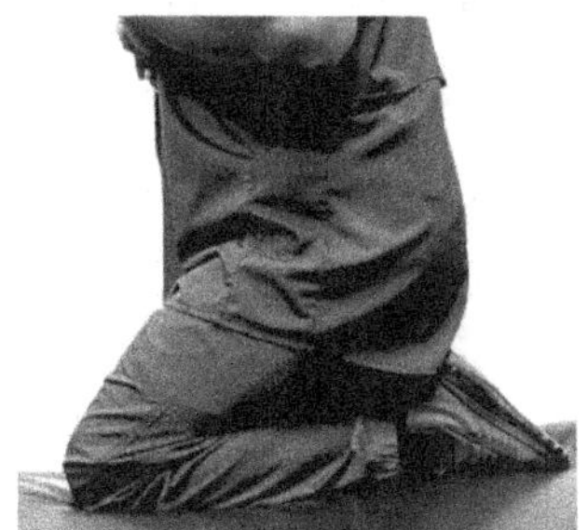

Books by Carson Robertson DC

Low Back Treatment Guide

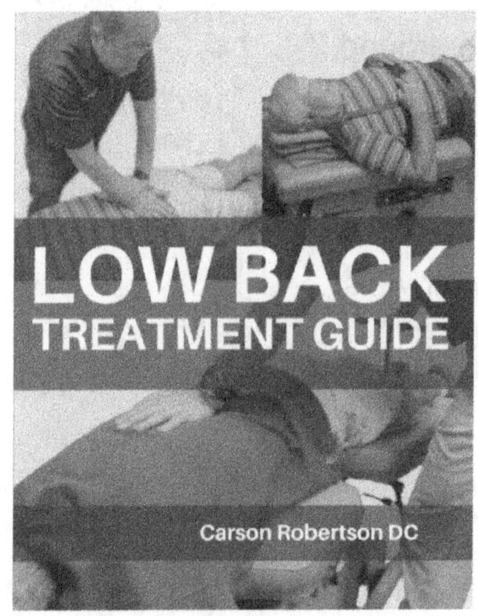

This book offers multiple conservative approaches to managing back pain at home and in the office. It provides several treatment options and strategies to improve your quality of life and eliminate debilitating back pain through a combination of non-invasive treatments and corrective exercise. After reading this book, you'll have the tools to take a more educated look in the mirror; to discover postural problems, dysfunctional movements, and daily habits that may be contributing to your condition. It would be misleading to promise that this book can "cure" your low back pain. What this book can do is help you manage your pain, improve your quality of life, and enjoy your recreational activities. You'll learn to be a better advocate for your own body, leading to a healthier and happier life.

Ultimate Knee Guide For Getting Rid of Pain & Avoiding Surgery: For Those with Grey Hair, Lots of Experience, & Some Wisdom

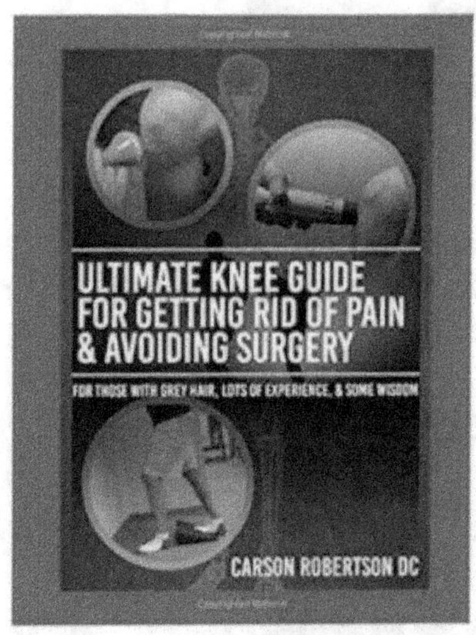

A guide to all conservative and medical treatments available to reduce your knee pain. A variety of knee conditions, home therapies, home products, and exercises are explained to educate and inform you of options available.Most people can successfully avoid knee surgery if they follow the correct treatments and exercise program. Unfortunately most people do not get the right treatments or recommendations, which leads them down the path to surgery. Have you talked to providers who are experts at knee rehabilitation? How do you know you are getting the best advice for your specific condition and where do you go to learn and educate yourself? Most cases of chronic knee pain are a slow development of increasing knee pain over time with subtle loss of function; and can be improved with the right therapy and treatments. Too many people make the mistake of having surgery first, and then going for rehabilitation. Maybe they should go for great rehab first and then surgery if absolutely needed.

Plantar Fasciitis Treatment Guide

People with plantar fasciitis become frustrated with the lack of clear answers, fluctuating foot pain, and various opinions. This complete guide reviews causes of plantar fasciitis, home therapies, home products, conservative treatments, medical treatments, alternative treatments, and provides effective exercises.

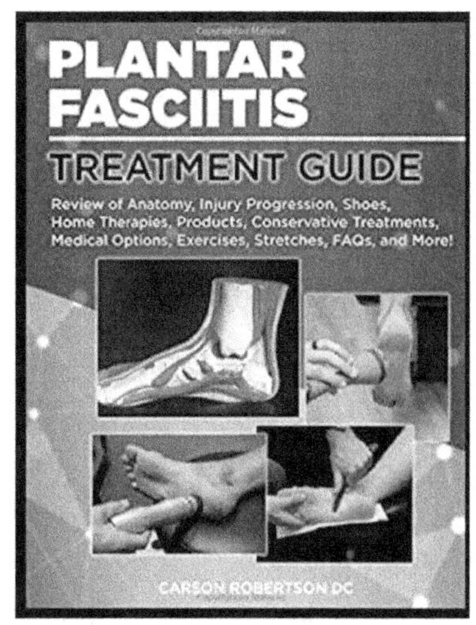

The book clearly explains and educates you on available options. Learn about plantar fasciitis, possible treatments, and home solutions in one book from someone who treats it every day. When do you ice vs heat? When should you consider orthotics or cortisone injections? Is a night splint worth the sleep loss? How big of a role do bone spurs play in heel pain? What are the most effective treatments for breaking up scar tissue and causing proper tissue healing? Most people will require a few different treatments to resolve their foot pain, but which ones provide the greatest benefit?

Elbow Pain Treatment Guide: Elbow Injuries & Treatments - Adults & Seniors

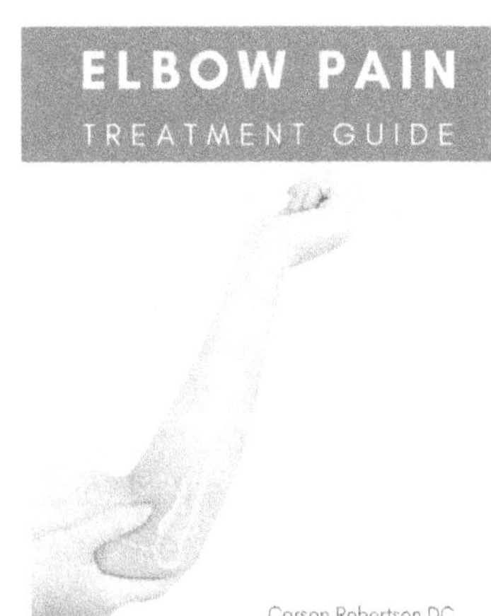

Most adult elbow injuries are the result of overuse and dysfunctional movement patterns. Although this book addresses both acute and chronic injuries, it focuses on the latter due to their high prevalence.

This book focuses on conservative therapies that can be performed at home or in the office for several elbow injuries. Because most elbow injuries don't occur in isolation, this book addresses these injuries within the larger framework of the upper extremity, movement patterns, past injuries, compensation patterns, and chronic repetitive injuries.

Most musculoskeletal injuries can be successfully treated or at worst case managed with a combination of physiotherapy and corrective exercise, especially treatments that focus on muscles, tendons, and ligaments.

Improve Your Game and Reduce Injuries: Simple Home Exercises & Stretches To Improve Your Golf Swing and Stay Pain Free

Golf doesn't pose some of the injury risks that high impact sports such as running or basketball do, playing the game with bad form can lead to injury. Although improper golf mechanics may not cause injuries in the short term, they most likely will catch up with the person at some point and possibly sideline him or her.

The purpose of this book is to connect the dots: to explain some of the differences between proper and improper golf mechanics, how improper movements are leading to injury, and most importantly, what can be done to fix them.

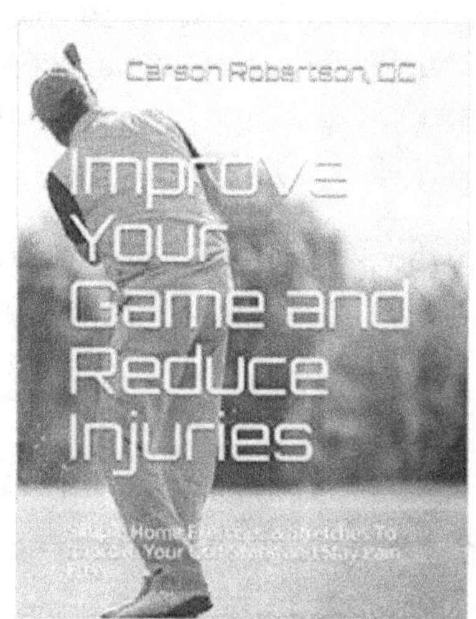

Hand & Wrist Treatment Guide For Adults

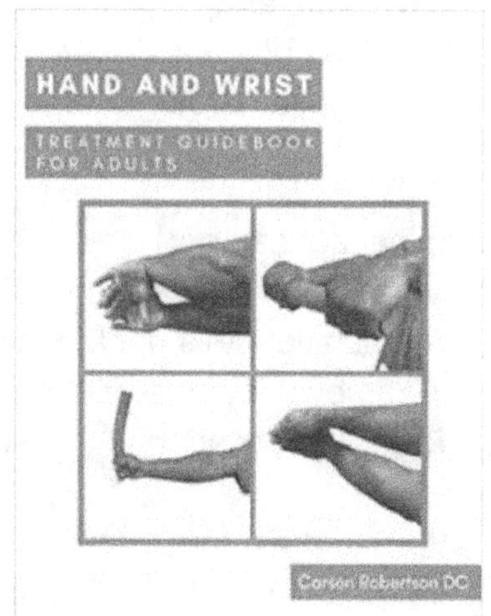

This book offers multiple conservative treatment approaches to improving and managing hand and wrist pain at home and in the office. Many patients require a combination of treatments to decrease pain and enhance tissue repair. The treatment guide provides several treatment options and strategies to eliminate your pain and get you back to your activities quickly.

This hand and wrist book provides multiple treatment strategies for those who want to do it on their own. It also covers the most effective office treatments, for those who need more help. More importantly, it describes treatment options for those who are not improving with basic office therapy. There are more options available than you think.

Upper Extremity Exercises for Adults & Seniors

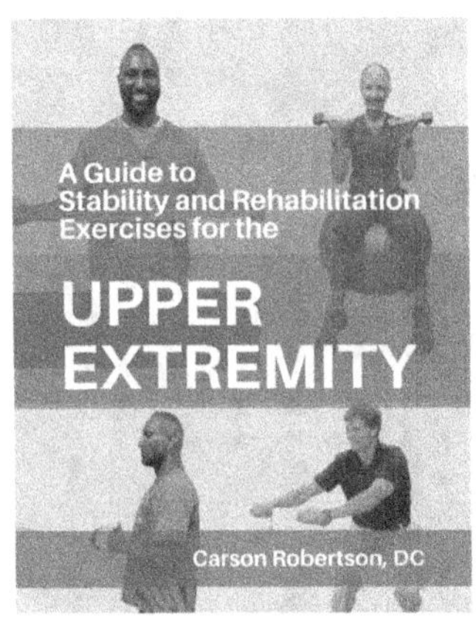

A variety of exercises to increase strength, flexibility, and range of motion for the upper extremity. It includes a variety of rehabilitation and strengthening exercises for adults and seniors to safely return from injury and enhance their functional abilities. This guide includes exercises that incorporate core and scapular strength with shoulder stabilization exercises to give adults an efficient set of progressive exercises to return from injury. It should be obvious an older body shouldn't be given the same exercises as the 20-year-old baseball player, so these exercises combine progressive stabilization exercises with functional abilities that adults can utilize to stay pain free and enjoy their daily activities. It includes the simpletest exercises to perform with an injury and ends with much harder exercises for the most motivated adults.

Stretch Series For Adults - With Average to Poor Flexibility

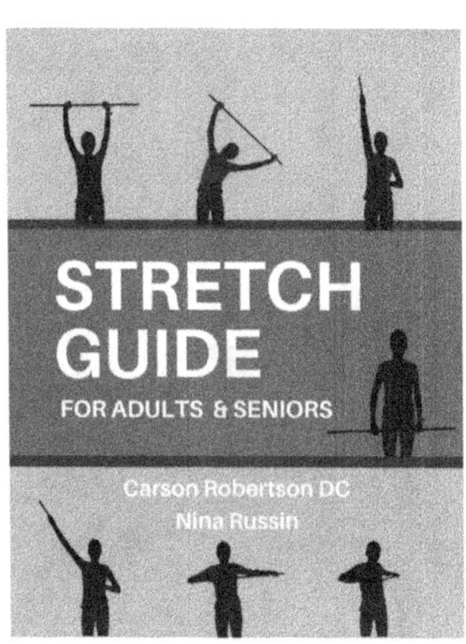

Stretching can be confusing for many, especially if their introduction was in high school gym class. Stretching should be comfortable, *not* painful. There are hundreds of ways to stretch the body, but the best stretches are the ones a person can do safely, comfortably, and consistently. The stretches you performed in high school are probably not feasible now, so this book combines multiple simple stretches for every region of the body. Be safe, consistent, and make progress to enhance your overall flexibility without causing injury.

Lower Extremity Exercises for Adults & Seniors

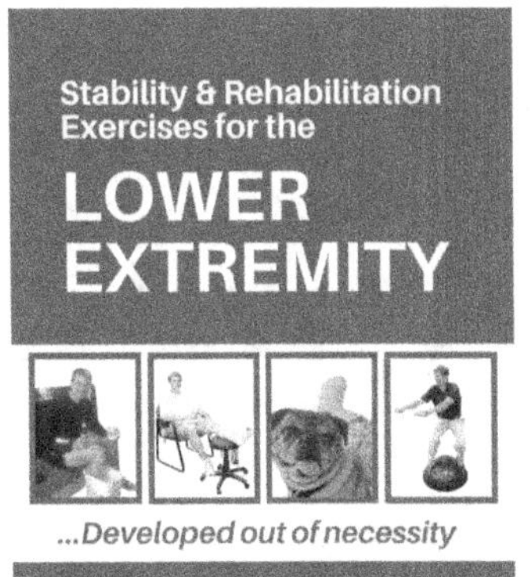

This exercise guide combines very simple to more advanced exercises for adults and those with gray hair. It includes modifications and stepping stone exercises starting from the most limited ability to more advanced. Ever gone to therapy and noticed you were given the exact same exercises as the teenager? Are those really the best exercises for an older body with some wear and tear on it? Functional abilities and goals are very different for those with a little gray hair, and this guide provides several options for accomplishing those functional goals with multiple variations of classic therapy exercises.

Core Exercises for Adults & Seniors

Quality of life and maintaining pain-free activities often involves working on the core and low back muscles. Many of the social media exercises seem too difficult or foreign for adults with gray hair to even attempt. This guide includes progressive stability and core exercises for those who want to be challenged.

The most effective strength training programs are those that require a minimal investment in equipment, and can be done anywhere. An exercise ball and a light weight is all you need.

The Swiss ball provides stimulus to the core muscles because it is inherently unstable. Basically, anything you can do on a weight bench can also be done on an exercise ball be it a bench press, military press, bicep curl, fly or row. The biggest difference between the bench and the ball is that the weight bench allows a person to isolate various parts of the body, whereas the ball, due to its instability, involves the entire body in every exercise. Because of this, you will want to begin with lighter weights, or in some cases, no weights at all.

Shoulder Pain Treatment Guide for Adults & Seniors

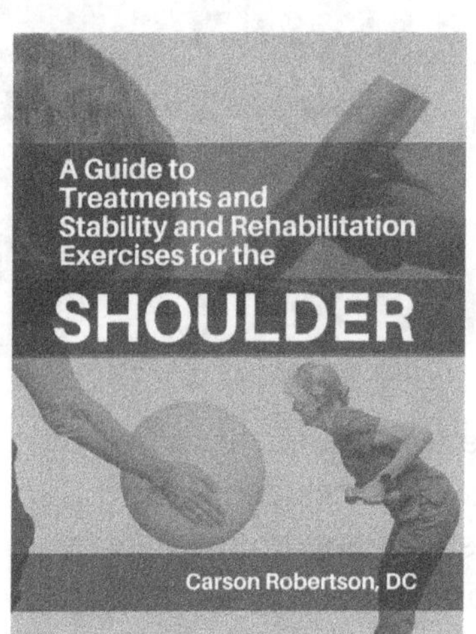

The advantage of a highly mobile shoulder joint is that it gives incredible range of motion and function. The disadvantage is that mobility comes at a cost of less structural protection, leading to increased risk of injury.

The purpose of this book is to explain where your pain came from and the best ways to resolve it at home and in the office. Common shoulder injuries include damage to the rotator cuff muscles (particularly the supraspinatus), impingement, labral tears, frozen shoulder and tendonitis or tendonosis, nerve entrapments, SICK Scapula, upper cross syndrome, thoracic outlet syndrome, and more.

Home and office treatment options are included to enhance your recovery. A variety of exercises are shown from the most basic to advanced. We have included many more than the basics to give you options to strengthen your shoulder and avoid future injuries.

Balance Exercises for Seniors

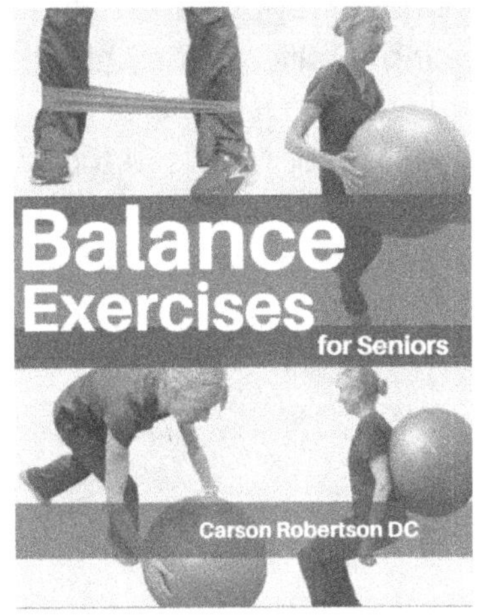

Most people do not notice their balance is slowly deteriorating over years because they never check it. Fortunately your balance can be improved by challenging yourself through a variety of standing and sitting on the ball exercises. This book contains simple balance and stability exercises for those getting started. The ball series starts with sitting on the ball to slowly build core and back stability safely. It progresses to exercises that slowly challenge people at their own pace.

The secret is to "challenge but not overwhelm." In the beginning simple exercises can improve your balance and decrease fall risks. For long term improvement, you need to teach the brain to listen to the lower extremity joints receptors and strengthen the stabilizer muscles.

Ball Exercises - Balance & Stability

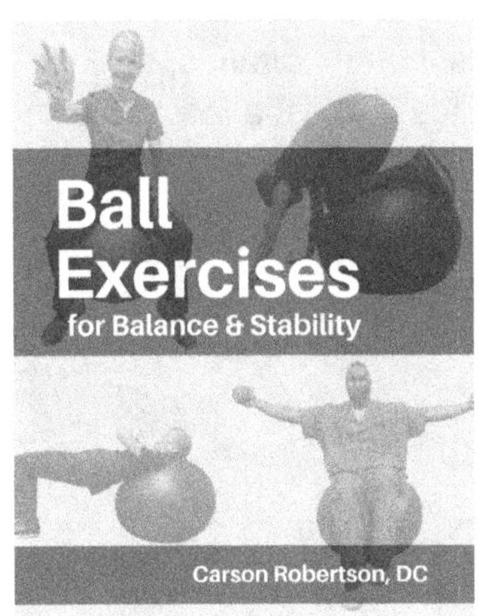

An exercise ball can be an entire workout and most people have never tried more than a few exercises on it. This book contains a variety of exercises for the entire body. It includes simple balance and stability exercises for those getting started. It contains a variety of exercises for the low back and core starting with basic exercises that progress to challenging push ups, planks, and mountain climbers. The series includes a variety of exercises sitting on the ball to slowly build core and back stability safely.

This book provides options on rehab exercises for a shoulder, elbow, or wrist. An exercise ball, bands, and a few weights produces a gym's worth of exercises to perform at home to safely get stronger and avoid injuries.

Max Goes to Sedona: Adventures of Max, Frances, & Lola

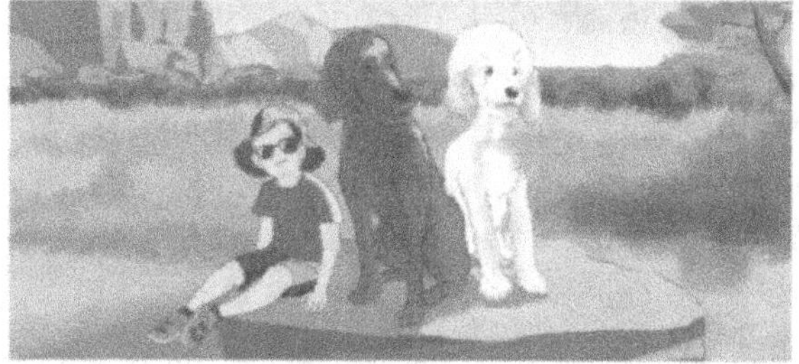

Max goes on a family vacation to Sedona, Arizona. He has a great weekend exploring trails with his best friends, Frances and Lola. The trio finds interesting wildlife as they hike the red dirt trails. They hang out at the pool and visit their first vineyard for Mom's birthday. This is the first of many adventures where Max explores his world with Frances and Lola by his side. He brings his parents along, too, for transportation.

Max Goes to the Zoo: Adventures of Max Frances, & Lola

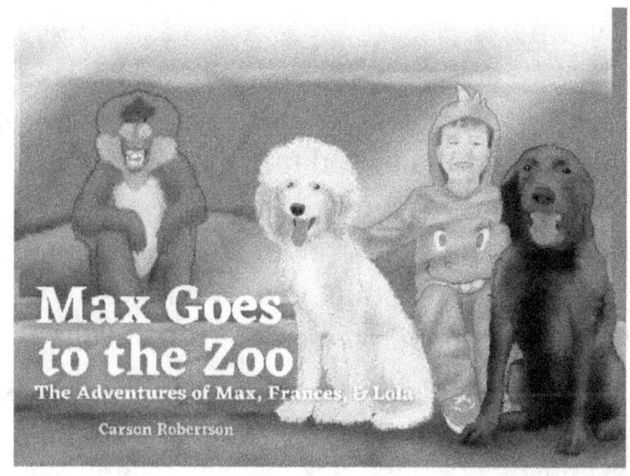

Three-year-old Max tells the story of his trip to the zoo with his best friends, Frances & Lola. He describes the adventure through his eyes, also pointing out what he likes about each animal. Roaring lions, lazy sloths, hungry giraffes, stinky camels, and rattling snakes are just a few stops along the way.

Max Gets Ready for Halloween: Adventures of Max, Frances, & Lola

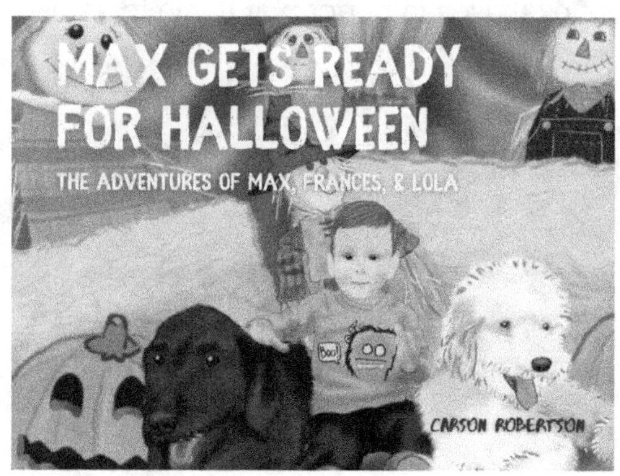

Three-year-old Max tells the story of his Halloweens with his best friends, Frances & Lola. Through his eyes he describes past Halloween costumes & activities. Max loves his family's tradition of going to Mother Nature's Farm to feed the animals, take a hayride, and pick out his pumpkins. Of course, Max also loves his matching costumes with Frances & Lola. Mom always has a theme.